Parkinson's Alternatives

Walk Better, Sleep Deeper and Move Consciously Solutions from Nature's Sensational Medicine

Kimberly Burnham, PhD
The Nerve Whisperer

Creating Calm Network Publishing Group

Published by The Creating Calm Network
Publishing Group, Spokane, Washington

ISBN: 978-1-937207-12-0

For reprint permissions and author
presentations

CCNPublishingGroup@gmail.com

TheBurnhamReview@juno.com

Walk Better, Sleep Deeper and Move Consciously

Are you one of the ten million people worldwide living with Parkinson's disease? Is someone you love losing their independence or their ability to walk due to Parkinson's?

Possibly you have found success in medications or surgery. Perhaps you are looking for other ways to decrease the tremors in your hands, so you can enjoy a dinner out with friends. Maybe you want to walk better or get rid of morning stiffness and get back into running. Maybe you are reading this book to learn some easy ways to balance your brain chemistry and feel more expressive, more focused, or to be more successful.

This book is also for Complementary and Alternative Medicine practitioners looking for ways to support recovery in clients with brain and nervous system issues.

Have you tried acupuncture for the symptoms of Parkinson's disease?

Have you been thinking about how Craniosacral therapy, Integrative Manual Therapy or Reiki could improve your life?

Maybe someone has talked to you about the benefits of Matrix Energetics, Emotional Freedom Technique's light tapping or even Nature's *Sensational Medicine*. Perhaps you have never heard of any of these things but you are searching for something that will help you feel better and are open to something new.

There is a saying, "You can't teach an old dog new tricks," but do you know the second part of the saying?

"The fastest way to become an old dog? ...
Stop learning new tricks."

Yes, some of these exercises may seem unconventional but before you decide, spend two minutes doing one of the many exercises, visualizations, or movements in *Parkinson's Alternatives: Walk Better, Sleep Deeper and Move Consciously; Solutions from Nature's Sensational Medicine*. Spend some time looking at the colors around you or reading the research from ancient Traditional Chinese Medicine or the latest article from Amy Cuddy, a Harvard professor who has found that two minutes of "Power Posing" or standing in a Wonder Woman or Superman posture can improve testosterone levels, literally making you a more powerful leader. Striking a two minute pose, standing or moving in a particular way also decreases cortisol levels, which makes you more adaptable and helps you feel less stressed.

Read the research linking dopamine to the energy of your gallbladder, even if it has been removed. In Acupuncture, the gallbladder meridian is associated with the color green. It is, along with the liver, a Wood Element. What if visualizing the color green flowing through your body, through your brain, through your liver and gallbladder could improve your control of movement, walking, or your facial expressions? Would it be worth spending two minutes a day?

What if visualizing yourself moving in a smooth controlled conscious way could help you in the real world to drive more safely, walk without falling and enjoy your family relationships more. Read the research on motor imagery, on using the mind to heal the brain, on the response of dopamine to physical exercises as well as imaginative rehabilitation exercises. Try out a few of the exercises.

Imagination is being able to see something before it is visible, before it is real in your life.

Would your life improve if you were more confident and compassionate or less angry and disappointed? What would change in the here and now if you could imagine a future with a full and independent life?

What if spending a few minutes a day, thinking about disgusting foods could improve your basal ganglia function. The basal ganglia is the part of the brain where surgically the deep brain stimulator is placed to suppress unwanted movements like ticks and tremors. What if your emotions could flow along the pathways that also light up the basal ganglia, making it possible for you to stand up, walk and turn as you navigate your world with more ease?

What do you have to let go of to harness the healing in your own hands and in your own mind? Are you consciously using touch to improve your independence, your movement, or your comfort?

As long as we are playing "What If", what if a few dollars for a book and a few minutes of your time each day could decrease some of the medical costs of Parkinson's?

The *Parkinson's Disease Foundation* estimates the combined direct and indirect cost of Parkinson's disease, including treatment, social security payments and lost income from inability to work, to be nearly $25 billion per year in the United States alone. Medication costs for an individual person with Parkinson's disease averages $2,500 a year, and therapeutic surgery can cost up to $100,000 dollars per patient.

Join me in the magical Matrix Energetics world of two points, fractal pathways, the homunculus in the brain, the gusto in disgust and more ways to heal from the field of *Sensational Medicine*. Use conscious sensation—touch, vision, insight, hearing, taste, smell, as well as internal sensation—to heal your brain, sleep deeper and to balance your dopamine levels.

Dopamine: the brain chemical of smooth voluntary movement, clarity of purpose and a sense of growth and development, serves to transmit nerve impulses and helps to regulate movement and emotions.

When dopamine, which can be an excitatory or inhibitory catecholamine [brain chemical or neurotransmitter] is functioning well you have feelings of pleasure and satisfaction as well as strong muscle control. Imbalanced dopamine shows up as the tremors of Parkinson's disease, the psychotic episodes and hallucinations of schizophrenia, tension headaches, poor intestinal function, addictions and attention disorders like autism, brain fog and attention deficit and hyperactivity disorder (ADHD).

As already mentioned, Dopamine is associated with the Traditional Chinese Medicine acupuncture meridian of the gallbladder, which is paired with the liver and considered to be a wood element, one of the five Chinese elements (Wood, Metal, Earth, Fire, and Water). Acupuncture (thin hair-like needles) or acupressure (fingertip pressure) provides a doorway into healing or a way to use sensations to heal. The gallbladder has also been linked to compassion, energy levels, cooperation, adaptability, organization, and self-expression.

How would the quality of your life change if you were more organized?

Sensations and the realm of *Sensational Medicine* includes the way you experience the world, the colors, shapes, textures, sounds, sights, tastes, smells and all the vibrations and energy that come to you from the world around you. Sensations can also relay information from one part of your body, say from the outside of your right fourth toe, to the brain. Internal sensations also include a sense of light, comfortable pressure under the right side of your lower rib cage, the home of your liver and gallbladder.

7

Associated with sensations, the gallbladder also governs your energy levels and awareness of the green and brown pigmented bile and gallbladder. In the ebb and flow of the Traditional Chinese Medicine clock, the gallbladder activity is heightened and most active from 11 pm to 1 am every night.

What time do you go to sleep? Are you sleeping deep and restfully by 11 pm?

Both the gallbladder and the liver are strongly connected to your parasympathetic nervous system, the "Rest and Digest" part of the automatic or autonomic nervous system. It is interesting to note that often Parkinson's disease tremors lessen at night. Throughout this book are exercises or ways for you to use this information—these connections—to heal.

To help you sleep deeper and heal more fully as you sleep, rest one hand over your lower right rib cage, mentally connecting that hand to your gallbladder and your liver, which sit just inside from the bones of the rib cage. Above the liver and gallbladder is the tough yet flexible diaphragm. Feel the diaphragm as it creates a lifting and lowering sensation within the rib cage enabling you to breathe in oxygen and exhale carbon dioxide, which you no longer need. What else can you draw into your life or exhale and release?

≈≈≈≈≈≈≈

Nature's *Sensational Medicine*

The aim of *Sensational Medicine* is to heal the sensory system with new activities. Remember ...."The fastest way to become an old dog? ... Stop learning new tricks."

So this year learn a new trick, observe a new sensation, or notice something old in a new way. These are ways to improve your brain health, your nervous system function, and decrease your pain while improving the quality of your life and the way you move and contribute to your community. Do something unique today to feel better, accomplish your goals and bring a smile to your face.

Try this right now: Pick something up every day and notice the shape, color, texture, sound, taste, smell, temperature, and consistency. Notice how the parts make up the whole and how it is connected to its surroundings. How is it similar or different from the other things around you? What changes in you when you truly see your natural environment and the people around you?

Here are exercises that help you to see others, your connections and relationships while noticing your surroundings. These activities connect you to the cycles and rhythms of life.

One purpose of vision is to see the support and resources available to you whether that is in the form of food from nature, a smile on a friend's face or a tree that brings beauty and shelter into your life.

What is the purpose of your sense of sound, taste, smell, and all the information, vibrations, and energy coming from the outside, meeting all of your internal sensations and creating meaning in your brain?

What is the purpose of your memory, of past learning, your sense of accomplishment in "The Now", and your hopes and images of a brighter, more colorful future?

Please enjoy these exercises, and most of all let them help you enjoy life and love more fully.

Kimberly Burnham, PhD, The Nerve Whisperer
Spokane, Washington KimberlyBurnhamPhD.com

Sensational Medicine and *Complementary and Alternative Medicine* Private Practice at St. Luke's Rehabilitation Institute, a small rehab hospital in the heart of Eastern Washington.

Amazon Author's Page
Amazon.com/Kimberly-Burnham/e/B0054RZ4A0

LinkedIn Profile: Linkedin.com/in/kimberlyburnham

≈≈≈≈≈≈≈

Other Books From
Kimberly Burnham, PhD, The Nerve Whisperer

Balancing the Sleep-Wake Cycle: Sleep Better, Learn Faster, Contribute More, and Enjoy Life to Its Fullest

Our Fractal Nature, A Journey of Self-Discovery and Connection, Psychology Meets Science

Live Like Someone Left The Gate Open

Parkinson's Alternatives: Walk Better, Sleep Deeper and Move Consciously, Solutions from Nature's Sensational Medicine.

Regain Your Balance: Ataxia Solutions from The Nerve Whisperer, Find Health and Healing in Six Complementary and Alternative Medicine Arenas

The Rhythm Cure, Diabetes Sensational Medicine Solutions, Reconnecting to the Cycle of Self-Awareness

Harnessing the Placebo Effect, It Is Not What you Think, It Is What You Expect

The Journey Home, One Woman's Bicycle Trips Across the US, Into Life

Anthologies From
Kimberly Burnham, PhD, The Nerve Whisperer

Pearls of Wisdom: 30 Inspirational Ideas to Live Your Best Life Now! with Jack Canfield, Marci Shimoff, Janet Attwod, Chris Attwood, and ...

No Mistakes!: How You Can Change Adversity into Abundance with Madisyn Taylor, Sunny Dawn Johnston, HeatherAsh Amara, Ann White and ...

Pebbles in the Pond: Transforming the World One Person at a Time (Wave One) with Christine Kloser, Ann White, Doreen G Fulton, Mary Dirksen, Denise Wade and ...

Tears to Triumph, Stories to Transform Your Life Today with Ann White, Doreen G Fulton, Mary Jane Giardi and ...

Bicycling for Food-Stories from the Intersection of Cycling, Food and Sustainability with Paul Burnham, Kathy Hansen, Victoria Carmona, Viviann Napp and ...

Music, Carrier of Intention in 49 Jewish Prayers with Elizabeth Goldstein, Ann White, Shefa Gold, Rami Shapiro, and ...

Healing Through Words with William Peters, Janet Caldwell, Ann White, Mary Dirksen, and ...

World Healing ~ World Peace Volume II: a poetry anthology with William Peters, Janet Caldwell, Ann White and ...

I Want My Poetry To . . . Volume II with The Anthological Poets, William S Peters, Monte Smith and ...

The Year of the Poet, 2014 monthly poetry book series from Inner Child Press and the Poetry Posse.

"I often say now I don't have any choice whether or not I have Parkinson's, but surrounding that non-choice is a million other choices that I can make." — Michael J. Fox

Walk Better, Sleep Deeper and Move Consciously, Contents

≈≈≈≈≈≈≈

Your Nervous System Can Heal & Serve You Better

Just a few years ago, when I asked a neurologist if the brain and spinal cord could heal and regenerate, he said "no" and in his world, maybe 20 years ago, that was true. Not particularly useful but in that time and space— true. The cool thing about today is a neurologist reading his or her own medical research literature is compelled to answer "yes, under certain circumstances." Here we will together explore those circumstances.

In this book I will explain what some of those healing circumstances are, and show you how to use information and sensations to speed up the healing process, so that you can walk around the neighborhood, confidently go out to eat, see the pyramids, and listen to the birds outside your window. In short, you will be given the tools to influence whatever you want to experience in your body, your nervous system and your life.

You might be saying to yourself, I don't believe this, there isn't any evidence, or it won't help me. The *Sensational Medicine* contained within this book can still meet your needs and can still help you. Placebo-controlled double-blind studies on information and sensation based medicine approaches like homeopathy and Matrix Energetics are few and far between, but as the *British Journal of Medicine* pointed out a few years ago, there are also no placebo-controlled double-blind studies on the value of parachutes for significant vertical drop but you would still be wise to have one on if you are jumping out of a plane.

If you are looking for ways to feel better, live a productive life, get up in the morning with the energy and the ability to take care of your personal needs before setting out on an exciting day in the world, you would be wise to explore *Sensational Medicine*.

≈≈≈≈≈≈≈

Part 1: So What is *Sensational Medicine*?

Sensational Medicine is the use of sensations, vibrations, energy and information as medicine. Information, vibration, and energy come to us through our senses. Homeopathy is perhaps the most common use of information in a healing way or Information Medicine. There are no medications, herbs, vitamins or nutrients in homeopathic remedies. What there is—is information in the form of a vibration or a pattern. When a person takes a homeopathic remedy they are putting new information into their body. This information interacts with the patterns of information, energy and matter already in play in the body.

New information interacting with an old pattern is a game changer.

In this book we will look at specific forms of information that can benefit people with a diagnosis of Parkinson's disease. Notice I said "people with a diagnosis of Parkinson's disease." I didn't say cure Parkinson's disease. If you are looking for a cure talk with your individual health-care practitioners. I didn't say cure Parkinson's disease, not because I am not allowed to but because this is nothing to do with the disease process and everything to do with people who could use some support. Is that you?

The philosopher, Plato encouraged, *"Be kind, for everyone you meet is fighting a hard battle."* Where in your life do you need more kindness? Where do you have kindness to give? This book shows you how to use information in many forms—pictures, words, sounds, touch, vibrations and frequencies—to be kind to yourself, your nervous system and those around you.

Other forms of information medicine contributing to the health and well being of millions of people include fields with names like Matrix Energetics, the Hawaiian Ho'oponopono, fractal homeomorphics, manual fractal patterning, reiki, and therapeutic touch.

≈≈≈≈≈≈≈

Letters and Words

What is the power of words? Does it matter if you are told by someone credible to you, "I have a number of clients who are living productive energetic lives with minimal symptoms of Parkinson's disease, ten plus years after diagnosis," or if they say, "You have Parkinson's disease, there is no cure and it will just get worse and worse." People have experienced both ways of looking at the label, for that is all it is—a label. By itself, it doesn't mean anything about your future, your prognosis, your ability to live the life you want.

People are devastated when told, "You have Parkinson's disease." Not because these words or letters are particularly devastating but because of all the information and meaning that has been assigned to them.

On the other hand when people are told "you have—Naiad Kiss Response or Spanks Iron Seaside," there is no devastation. These are the same letters, but they are formed into different words and more importantly they carry information and meaning that is vastly different from "Parkinson's Disease."

What are words but carriers of information? Words, written, read, spoken, and heard, each form a pillar of *Sensational Medicine*. What words and sounds are you paying attention to? What words are you accepting as true, as real, as your future? What are you saying as every cell in your body listens?

≈≈≈≈≈≈≈

Exercise: Morning Words

1. For the next seven days, notice what the first 10 words out of your mouth are when you get up in the morning. Do you always say the same thing? Do you always talk to the same people? Are the first words you say over the phone? Do you ever talk to a stranger first thing in the morning?

Just notice what you say and how the noticing changes you and what you say.

2. For the next seven days, notice who asks you, "How are you?"

What do you say as every cell in your body listens?

≈≈≈≈≈≈≈

Results, Problems and Road Blocks

I have used *Sensational Medicine* to help myself overcome neurological disorders, genetic conditions, chronic pain issues, autoimmune disease and I have helped thousands of clients do the same. *Sensational Medicine* is easy to understand, quick to take effect and powerful. It is also hard to believe and that I believe gets in the way of most people taking control of their health and wellness.

The problems is most people get fooled by people claiming there is only one way to heal or worse that there is nothing you can do or blame the disease and dysfunction on the aging process. I am one of the people who feel better and function better as I get older. My vision is better than when I was forty and better than when I was 12 and started wearing glasses.

You are probably like many of my clients when they first started using *Sensational Medicine*, someone twisted their arm, pushed them, begged them to do something besides the conventional approaches they had been using without success. Or you might be like the people who grew tired of being told there is nothing you can do and set out to find something that can improve symptoms and decrease pain.

When confronted with a diagnosis of Parkinson's disease most people in their heart are not surprised, they know something has been wrong for a while but they get overwhelmed by the pile of information that says they will get worse and worse, eventually becoming a burden on their family, unable to take care of even basic needs themselves.

It doesn't have to be this way. You do have choices. They are just not conventional and many are not supported by placebo-controlled double-blind studies. *Sensational Medicine* approaches are back up by something even better, caring practitioners and coaches, thousands of happy, healthy, comfortable clients and the magical science of quantum physics.

Sometimes when people hear the words—quantum physics—they worry that it will be too complicated, that if they don't understand the detailed science in the background, the technique or approach won't work for them. In much the same way that a light bulb allows you to read at night whether or not you know that the electricity came from coal burning, solar panels, or a windmill, *Sensational Medicine* tools and techniques work regardless of whether you understand, how that information was created, where it came from or how it was delivered to you. You just have to make use of it. Do a few of the exercises and see what it can do for you.

Millions of people have benefitted from acupuncture or craniosacral therapy without having any idea how it works on the mind, body and spirit. What they usually know is that their friend got rid of migraines with craniosacral therapy or an acupuncturist helped their brother with back pain. They try it and then they know how much it can help them feel better and achieve the goals they want in their life.

I find that in reaching a healthy lifestyle the biggest stumbling block is: not having the commitment to begin, because once you have begun you feel the results and see the changes as does everyone around you.

There are millions of people in every part of the world, including Nebraska that didn't let fear of failure or the idea that people might make fun of them interfere with trying it out. They didn't let any of the stumbling blocks stop them and here we will discuss just a few of the results they got.

≈≈≈≈≈≈≈

"Attention is the way social primates measure status. It is highly rewarding because it causes the release of brain chemicals such as dopamine and endorphins." —Keith Henson.

Part 2: The Power Pose of Dopamine and Brain Health

"Don't fake it till you make it. Fake it till you become it," says Amy Cuddy, Harvard Business School professor. In a *TED Talk* she notes brain and body chemistry changes within two minutes of taking a power pose—think of the way Wonder Woman or Superman would stand, feet apart, hands on your hips.

Our bodies change our minds and our minds can change our behavior. Our behavior can change our outcomes and even our physiology, according to Cuddy, who has shown that standing or sitting for two minutes in an open posture can significantly increases testosterone, which is the assertiveness and dominance hormone. This open posture also decreases cortisol, which means you are less stressed.

It is easy. You need your body and two minutes to significantly change your life for the better.

"Body language shapes who you are but what is surprising, when it comes to power, is that the body also shapes the mind." Dana Carney (UC-Berkeley) and Amy Cuddy, both experimental social psychologists, have conducted research showing that adopting these postures—"power posing"—actually causes people to become more powerful. "After sitting or standing, alone in a room, in a high-power pose for just two minutes, participants in our experiments resembled powerful people—emotionally, cognitively, behaviorally, and even physiologically."

"They felt more powerful, were more willing to take risks, presented their ideas with greater confidence and enthusiasm, performed better in demanding situations, and experienced significant increases in testosterone—a hormone linked to assertiveness—and significant decreases in cortisol—a hormone linked to stress. In other words—two minutes of preparatory power posing optimizes the brain to function well in high-stakes challenges."

And really what aspect of your life is not a high stake challenge? Where in your life could you benefit from more power, greater confidence, and better performance?

More research follows but here are the exercises for balancing brain chemistry and improving your performance and enjoyment of life, regardless of a diagnosis.

≈≈≈≈≈≈≈

Exercise: Power Posing for Balancing Dopamine

Do any or all of these exercises on a daily basis for two minutes at a time.

1. Stand for two minutes in the Wonder Woman or Superman power pose: Feet apart (wider than your

shoulders) with your hands on your hips, head up and chest out slightly. While Amy Cuddy didn't measure changes in dopamine, she did find an increase in confidence and risk-taking behavior, which is associated with dopamine. I believe the research indicates this exercise can help balance dopamine levels. Lowering your cortisol levels, means you are less stressed. Less stress and a more powerful feeling often mean your tremors and symptoms are lessened.

2. Stand for two minutes in the Wonder Woman or Superman power pose: Feet apart (wider than your shoulders) with your hands on your hips, head up and chest out slightly. Do this for two minutes before meals as you think about what you are going to be eating. What is the color, texture, taste and smell of the food you are about to eat? Where did it come from? Who grew or produced it? Who prepared it for you? What is your favorite part of the meal? This kind of mindfulness combined with a more powerful feeling and less stress improves digestion, improves your absorption of the iron, protein and fats you need to produce dopamine and heal your brain.

I had a nutrition teacher at Sutherland-Chan Massage School in Toronto Canada, who said, "You can get more nutrition from a hot dog with friends than an organic gourmet meal with people you hate." Your level of stress and level of consciousness as you eat combines to significantly influence your digestion and absorption of needed nutrients.

3. Consciously walk with long strides. Consciously increase the distance between your feet as you walk for two minutes. This can be outside on a sunny winter's day; inside the familiarity of your home; in a quite soothing library; or the hustle and bustle of a shopping mall.

In Parkinson's disease, a loss of dopamine producing cells in the midbrain (substantia nigra) leads to a shuffling gait or short steps. Integrative Manual Therapy and acupuncture or acupressure, both have been shown to improve stride length and there is lots of research to show the benefits of walking for people with Parkinson's disease.

What if walking like you have strong dopamine producing cells actually increased their ability to produce dopamine? I don't know the answer to that question yet, but what I know is that consciously increasing your stride length results in improved walking and balance for some people. It has also decreased back and hip pain.

4. Dopamine is associated with Traditional Chinese Medicine's Gallbladder Meridian. A stretch for the gallbladder meridian and an activation exercise for the energy that flows along the meridian is to sit on the floor. Stretch your legs out straight to the side as wide apart as

possible, creating a V shape with your hips at the narrow end and each foot at the wide end.

Note: Stretching should always be pain-free. Do not stretch through the pain. Stretch to a comfortable range and then imagine yourself stretching to the end range. Little by little you may find yourself stretching comfortably farther and farther.

Fold your fingers together so your palms are facing away from your chest as you breathe. Fingers together, palms facing away, stretch your arms over your head. Then bend forward to the side and try to touch your toes with the palms of your hands. Do this on each side. As you breathe deeply in and out, notice any changing sensation in your legs. The liver meridian runs along the inner legs while the gallbladder meridian runs along the outer side of the legs. There is more about the gallbladder and liver meridians later.

By combining this exercise with medical research on motor imagery (read more about it in the research and references section) I came up with this question: What if you just started by imagining yourself in this position, visualizing yourself stretching in this way? Imagine how your shoulders and hips would feel. What signals would be sent from your arms and legs to your brain? How would the position change the feel of your clothing on your skin? Which muscles would be most stretched?

How would the increased flexibility influence your walking as you leave the house in the morning?

Imagine what can change and how rewarding just imagining yourself doing this stretch would be. Imagine the benefits until you can do the stretch fully with your physical body. In other words, "Fake it, till you become it," and see changes immediately.

5. Two muscles are associated with the Acupuncture's Wood elements (liver and gallbladder) and therefore with dopamine. The anterior deltoid muscle at the shoulder and popliteus at the back of the knee are associated with the gallbladder and dopamine, while the pectoralis major sternal segment of the chest muscles and rhomboids at the back of the shoulders are associated with the liver and norepinephrine. You can activate these muscles by stretching your arms and shoulders as well as your legs and knees.

Again note: Stretching should always be pain-free. Do not stretch through the pain. Stretch to a comfortable range and then imagine yourself stretching to the end range. Little by little you may find yourself stretching comfortably farther and farther.

For the deltoid muscle: Stand at edge of a wall or in doorway facing perpendicular to wall. Position the palm of your right hand on the surface of wall slightly lower than your shoulder. Bend elbow slightly. Turn your body away from the positioned arm. Hold stretch for 30 seconds or so. Repeat with opposite arm.

For the pectoralis major stretch: Stand with one forearm resting on the side of the door frame with the elbow flexed 90 degrees and shoulder abducted (away from the body) 90 degrees. Keep your forearm on the side of the door frame as you step forward slightly until a stretch is felt across your chest. Turn your head away from the side that is being stretched to deepen the stretch.

As with above, what if you just started by imagining yourself doing these stretches first thing in the morning or in the evening before you fall asleep. Imagine how your back and shoulders would feel. What changes would there be in the circulation to the big muscles of your arms and legs and to your brain just by imagining yourself doing these stretches? What would change in the colors and shapes you noticed around you if you could turn your head with more ease? How would the increased flexibility influence what you bought at the store as you walked with more confidence?

Imagine what can change and how rewarding just imagining yourself doing these stretch would be. Imagine the benefits until you can do the stretch fully with your physical body. In other words, "Fake it, till you become it," and see changes immediately.

6. The emotions associated with the gallbladder and the liver are anger and compassion. Imagine yourself

physically expressing your anger in a constructive way. Imagine yourself in an act of compassion. What is your body posture of compassion? What if you were an actor in an improvisation group and you had to act out or express anger or compassion? What if you were playing Charades, how would you express the word, compassion? Use visualization to help you express and harness rather than suppress these two emotions.

7. The following two minute position comes from *Advanced Strain and Counterstrain* by Sharon W Giammatteo and from the field of Integrative Manual Therapy. It is designed to improve blood flow through the legs. Place one hand over the left front of the hip and the other hand resting on the back of the neck. Sit on the edge of a chair with your legs out in front of you. Spread your legs so that there is about 30 degrees between your right and left leg. Keep the knees straight. Turn your feet and ankles out slightly so that your toes point away from the center of our body. Lean forward slightly so there is more flexion at the hips and then rest your hands on your knees. Relax the leg muscles as much as possible and breathe slowly for two minutes.

As I mentioned at the beginning of this section try out one or two of these exercises. Consciously notice what changes in how you feel and more. You may want to get the help of an athletic trainer or physical therapist with these stretches. Feel free to take this information to your therapist or trainer, so they can support your healing process more fully.

≈≈≈≈≈≈≈

Overview of Posture, Movement and Power Posing Research and References

If you are interested, read more of the research and reference material on power posing, using your body to affect your brain, motor imagery and proprioception [a sense of where you are in space].

You can see Amy Cuddy's *TED Talk* on power posing, changes in testosterone and cortisol from adopting a two minute posture at Ted.com/talks/amy_cuddy_your_body_language_shapes _who_you_are.html

For a picture of some of the Advanced Strain and Counterstrain positions see an article by Lissa Wheeler. (2004) "*Advanced Strain Counterstrain.*" Massage Therapy Journal 43 Winter (4): [Full Text] www.amtamassage.org/uploads/cms/documents/advanc edStrainCounterstrain.pdf

This is what Sharon W. Giammatteo says about improving circulation to the legs. "This technique will affect circulation of the leg, including arterial flow, venous return and lymphatic drainage. This technique is excellent for soft tissue dysfunction, including myofascial dysfunction, scar tissue, protective muscle spasm, and other less circulatory-specific problems." —Giammatteo, T. and S. Weiselfish-Giammatteo (1997). *Integrative manual therapy for the autonomic nervous system and related disorders: utilizing advanced strain and counterstrain technique.* Berkeley, Calif., North Atlantic Books. This book is designed for physical therapists and massage therapists to use the techniques with their clients.

Here are a few quotes on the topic of movement, posture, and motor imagery from researchers.

"The ability to walk safely without falling and in an energy efficient manner significantly influences children and adults' quality of life and function. There are many reasons for balance problems and gait dysfunction, including injury, pain, neurological damage and vascular impairment. Integrative Manual Therapy, Osteopathic Manual Medicine, Massage Therapy, Cranial Therapy, Muscle Energy, Strain and Counterstrain, Acupuncture and Qigong are some of the most effective ways to increase mobility. These complementary and alternative therapies (CAM) often lead to pain-free efficiency in walking, running and movement. — Burnham Kimberly. PhD. IMTC. LMT (2009). "Using Manual Therapy to Improve Gait Function in Neurodegenerative Disorders." *Journal of the Integrative Manual Therapy Association* August, 3(2)

One theory of emotional expression dates back to 1906 and "holds that facial muscles act as ligatures on facial blood vessels and thereby regulate cerebral blood flow, which, in turn, influences subjective feeling." The theory, developed by Israel Waynbaum, a French physician, hypothesizes "the subjective experience of emotions as following facial expression rather than preceding it." —Zajonc, R. B. (1985). "Emotions and facial expression." *Science* 230(4726): 608-687.

Perhaps this explains why laughter is such a positive influence on health. It begs the question, "Do we laugh because we are happy or do we laugh so our brains will get better blood flow and then we will feel happy?"

"One of the most remarkable capacities of the mind is its ability to simulate sensations, actions, and other types of experience. A mental simulation process that has attracted recent attention from cognitive neuroscientists and sport psychologists is motor imagery or the mental rehearsal of actions without engaging in the actual physical movements involved." —Moran, A., A. Guillot, et al. (2012). "Re-imagining motor imagery: building bridges between cognitive neuroscience and sport psychology." *Br J Psychol* 103(2): 224-247.

"Motor imagery has recently gained attention as a promising new rehabilitation method for patients with neurological disorders." —Heremans, E., P. Feys, et al. (2011). "Motor imagery ability in patients with early- and mid-stage Parkinson disease." *Neurorehabil Neural Repair* 25(2): 168-177.

"Performance impairment is a consequence of fatigue, but alterations on perception and mental activity may also occur. Muscle fatigue, unlike fatigue induced by prolonged exercise, does not elicit mental fatigue and therefore does not alter motor imagery accuracy." — Guillot, A., M. Haguenauer, et al. (2005). "Effect of a fatiguing protocol on motor imagery accuracy." *Eur J Appl Physiol* 95(2-3): 186-190.

"Evidence from previous studies has suggested that motor imagery and motor action engage overlapping brain systems. As a result of this observation that motor imagery can activate brain regions associated with actual motor movement, motor imagery is expected to enhance motor skill performance and become an underlying principle for physical training in sports and physical rehabilitation." —Baeck, J. S., Y. T. Kim, et al. (2012). "Brain activation patterns of motor imagery reflect plastic changes associated with intensive shooting training." *Behav Brain Res* 234(1): 26-32.

Hernandez-Reif and Ironson wrote, "Women with breast cancer are at risk for elevated depression, anxiety, and decreased natural killer (NK) cell number. Stress has been linked to increased tumor development by decreasing NK cell activity." After the massage therapy study, they concluded, "women with Stage 1 and 2 breast cancer may benefit from thrice-weekly massage therapy for reducing depressed mood, anxiety, and anger and for enhancing dopamine, serotonin, and NK cell number and lymphocytes". —Hernandez-Reif, M., G. Ironson, et al. (2004). "Breast cancer patients have improved immune and neuroendocrine functions following massage therapy." *J Psychosom Res* 57(1): 45-52.

"Pleasure can serve cognition, productivity and health, but simultaneously promotes addiction and other negative behaviors, i.e., motivational toxicity. It is a complex neurobiological phenomenon, relying on reward circuitry or limbic activity. These processes involve dopaminergic signaling. Moreover, endorphin and endogenous morphinergic mechanisms may play a role. Natural rewarding activities are necessary for survival and appetitive motivation, usually governing beneficial biological behaviors like eating, sex and reproduction." —Esch, T. and G. B. Stefano (2004). "The neurobiology of pleasure, reward processes, addiction and their health implications." *Neuro Endocrinol Lett 25(4): 235-51.* [Full Text]
http://www.nel.edu/pdf_/NEL250404R01_Esch-Stefano_p_.pdf

≈≈≈≈≈≈≈

Part 3: Using the Mind / Emotions to Heal the Brain
(Caring, Creativity, Frontal Lobe)

This section contains a series of exercises known as *Using the Mind to Heal the Brain*. Here we will look at the relationship between certain areas of the brain and particular emotions or expressions.

For example, there is a link between Caring, Creativity and the Frontal Lobe. What this means is that if someone has a car accident and hits their forehead on the windshield causing a brain injury to the frontal lobe or the part of the brain behind the forehead, there are a number of ways to address this injury and recover brain health.

≈≈≈≈≈≈≈

Exercise: Avocadoes, Olive Oil and Cashews for Brain Health

One lifestyle change is to eat brain healthy foods like the essential fatty acids in avocadoes, olive oil and cashews. The frontal lobe houses your cognitive ability, so doing activities like crossword puzzles or learning a new language also improve frontal lobe function.

The relationship with caring and creativity means that another doorway into brain health is available through putting yourself in a position where caring, compassion and empathy are required, such as taking care of a pet or volunteering at a nearby soup kitchen. Doing activities which express a caring attitude improves brain function as well as boosting creativity and lifting the haze of brain fog. On the other hand engaging in creative activities, creating art work, writing a poem, or planning and planting a garden has the added benefit of increasing learning and attention as well as enhancing compassion and frontal lobe function.

Imagine a cube with several doorways, marked Creativity, Caring, Frontal lobe function, Learning and Attention. Entering through any doorway improves all of the functions, including brain health, emotional function and thought processes. Each doorway leads to Mind-Body-Spirit health.

So what are the brain structures, emotions and behaviors that are an expression of dopamine balance? What activities can you do to improve brain chemistry?

≈≈≈≈≈≈≈

Exercise: Improve Cognitive Function, Keep Your Mind Sharp

Caring: Think about, plan and then do something that requires caring—caring for someone or something.

Imagine yourself in a caring situation. What is your posture like? What does your back feel like? Who is smiling at you?

Creativity: Think about, plan and carry out a creative project —a piece of art work, a poem, a piece of music.

Imagine creating a gift for someone. Imagine how they will look at you when you give them something you have made for them. Just imagine then do it if you want.

Frontal Lobe Function: Your brain thrives on novelty, on doing something new or solving a puzzle. Do something new today.

≈≈≈≈≈≈≈

Dopamine Balance, Using the Mind to Heal the Brain

Dopamine is associated with the Traditional Chinese Medicine Gallbladder meridian. The emotion of anger is related both to Acupuncture's Wood elements: Liver and Gallbladder as well as to dopamine imbalances.

Imagine a cube shaped house with brain chemistry, especially dopamine balance on one wall. Anger on another wall and the liver and gallbladder on the third side. The fourth side is the substantia nigra in the midbrain at the top of the brainstem and the basal ganglia.

These are the two brain structures most affected by dopamine balance. Dopamine is produced in the substantia nigra and then flows to the basal ganglia where it helps you suppress unwanted movements like tremors and ticks. Dopamine balance also enhances your ability to interact with the reality around you, without hallucinations.

Imagine that the whole house is green or brown, the colors associated with the gallbladder and liver in acupuncture.

≈≈≈≈≈≈≈

Imagine Visualize

Consider for a moment the difference between visualization, imagination and hallucination. Visualization is the conscious conjuring of an image in your mind's eye. It moves information from your conscious mind to your subconscious while at the same time allows you access to subconscious information.

Imagination is the ability to see what is not yet visible. When you imagine a positive thing for yourself in the future you create an expectation and that expectation influences brain chemistry. The placebo effect for example is the interaction between the story you tell yourself about how something will affect you and the story you believe from a healthcare professional. Since we don't know what the future will bring, it makes sense to imagine, predict and visualize positive things for ourselves.

Hallucinations on the other hand are not consciously created, are confusing and often frightening. It is the lack of consciousness that the problem. If I want to imagine a delicious Thanksgiving dinner with beloved friends and family there is no downside. The problem begins when images and experiences lurk about without consciousness of reality, time and space.

We could of course have a whole discussion about what is real and what is time and space in Newtonian physics and in the quantum world but the main point here is that awareness, relationship to self and others and consciousness are all very different in a hallucination compared with a visualization or something that you imagine consciously.

≈≈≈≈≈≈≈

Reach Out for What You Want

There is research indicating that for your brain it is easier to reach out for what you want than to let go of what you don't want. Applied to visualization, imagery and hallucinations, the research would suggest that it is easier to consciously create positive visualizations for yourself than to let go of or get rid of the hallucinations. Indications are that once you establish a visualization, guided imagery, or motor imagery practice the hallucinations or bad dreams will lessen on their own.

You may be interested to know that people with Parkinson's disease (too little dopamine) are more engaged by the placebo effect while people with schizophrenia (too much dopamine) are less engaged by the placebo effect.

≈≈≈≈≈≈≈

Exercises: Pick a Doorway

In this case imagine that each side of the cube can be balanced and improved by going through one of the doorways. Here are several things you can do to improve brain chemistry, dopamine balance, anger management, liver and gallbladder health as well as substantia nigra and basal ganglia function.

1. Eat cashews. They are high in nut fats and proteins, which help support brain function. They are also high in natural iron, which is a precursor to dopamine and important in sustaining red blood cell production and the oxygen carrying capacity of your blood. Leafy green and red vegetables are also high in iron and supportive of health in general as well as liver and gallbladder health.

2. Check into Community Support Agriculture (CSA) programs in your area to see how you can get fruits and vegetables that sustain you and your environment. Summer of 2013 I rode my bicycle 3000 miles across the

United States in support of sustainable agriculture and food justice. Follow my ride at https://www.youtube.com/watch?v=S9nZNVnDGLg

3. Get help with anger management through visualization, psychotherapy, exercises, walking, doing things that bring you pleasure, etc.

4. Consider what makes you angry. What helps you resolve feelings of anger? Practice taking a new perspective on the situation or relationship. How can you see things from a different perspective that will change how you feel about the world and the people around you? What do you do every day to improve your mood?

5. Play Charades or imagine that you are playing Charades. How would you physically express anger or its flip side, forgiveness, compassion, or empathy? What do these words look like or how would you move? Imagine how a friend or family member would express these words in a game of Charades.

Here are some movies, quotes and sayings that you can use in a real or imagined game of Charades.

Movies:
The Upside of Anger
Anger Management
Colors of Compassion

Love! Valour! Compassion!
Matrix of Compassion

iPhone App: *Angry Birds*

Sayings or quotes:

"Anger is a short madness." **—Horace (65-8 BC)**

"Exaggeration is truth that has lost its temper." **—Kahlil Gibran (1883-1931)**

"Fire in the heart sends smoke into the head." **—German Proverb**

"If you are patient in one moment of anger, you will escape a hundred days of sorrow." **—Chinese Proverb**

"If you kick a stone in anger you will hurt your foot." **—Korean saying**

"Postpone today's anger until tomorrow." **—Tagalog (Filipino) saying**

"Forgiveness is the fragrance the violet sheds on the heel that has crushed it." **—Mark Twain**

"Once a woman has forgiven her man, she must not reheat his sins for breakfast." **—Marlene Dietrich**

"It's easier to ask forgiveness than it is to get permission."
—**Grace Hopper**

"The weak can never forgive. Forgiveness is the attribute of the strong." —**Mahatma Gandhi**

"The dew of compassion is a tear." —**Lord Byron**

"If you want others to be happy, practice compassion. If you want to be happy, practice compassion." —**Dalai Lama**

6. Rest comfortably with one hand on your liver and gallbladder area (lower right side of the rib cage) and the other hand resting on the back of your head over the area of midbrain where the substantia nigra is located and is an access point for the basal ganglia. Connect the two areas in your mind for a few minutes. From Matrix Energetics comes the idea of the "Two Point Technique" and from Integrative Manual Therapy comes NeuroFascial Process or the One Hand Here, One Hand There Self-Care Approach.

7. Spend time looking at, wearing and drawing with the color green or brown. Notice what is in your house or surroundings that is made of wood. Notice the details and variations in the wood or green item.

Green is the color associated with the liver and gallbladder which are the wood elements in acupuncture.

8. Think of forgiveness as the flip side of anger. Spend a few minutes every day forgiving someone. This forgiveness could be for something small, for example, if someone takes too long to provide a service to you at a restaurant or a car wash. It could be something major that has been weighing on you for years. Today is the day to let go of the anger and embrace forgiveness, not only to make the world a better place but to make your brain and body a healthier place.

Each of these exercises is a doorway into a healthier brain, liver/gallbladder and emotional state. Each one influences the other.

≈≈≈≈≈≈≈

Some Research on Dopamine, Anger, Fear, Anxiety, Physical and Emotional Pain

"The associations reported in this article suggest that the 9-repeat allele of the dopamine transporter is associated with angry-impulsive personality traits, independent of any link to mood disorder or borderline personality disorder (BPD) in depressed patients. This could form the basis of a dopaminergic neurobiological model of angry-impulsive personality traits." —Joyce, P. R., P. C. McHugh, et al. (2009). "Relationships between angry-impulsive personality traits and genetic polymorphisms of the dopamine transporter." *Biol Psychiatry* 66(8): 717-721.

"Although the biological basis of trait anger, anger expression, and forgiveness are not well understood, there has been growing evidence that anger-related dispositions are heritable and associated with genetic polymorphisms. These findings suggest a possible relationship between anger expression styles and forgiveness traits and dopaminergic dysfunction." — Kang, J. I., K. Namkoong, et al. (2008). "Association of DRD4 and COMT polymorphisms with anger and forgiveness traits in healthy volunteers." *Neurosci Lett* 430(3): 252-257.

"Dopamine plays an important role in fear and anxiety modulating a cortical brake that the medial prefrontal cortex exerts on the anxiogenic output of the amygdala and have an important influence on the trafficking of impulses between the basolateral (BLA) and central nuclei (CeA) of amygdala ... It is suggested that D1- and D2-dopamine receptors in the amygdala may have a differential role in the modulation of anxiety. The possibility is discussed that D1 receptors participate in danger whereas D2 receptors have a role in setting up adaptive responses to cope with aversive environmental stimuli." —de la Mora, M. P., A. Gallegos-Cari, et al. (2010). "Role of dopamine receptor mechanisms in the amygdaloid modulation of fear and anxiety: Structural and functional analysis." *Prog Neurobiol* 90(2): 198-216.

"Brain scans are clearly showing there is relatively little difference between physical pain and social pain (Eisenberger and Lieberman, 2004). If social pain has evolved much like hunger, thirst, or any other form of pain – as a signal to change behavior – and, as in the case of hunger or thirst, if the social pain goes unheeded it takes a serious toll on mind and biology and becomes increasingly difficult to overcome, what can social cognitive neuroscience tell us about the key drivers of social pain (and pleasure) in the workplace and particularly from the standpoint of workplace status, relatedness, and fairness.

In the same regard, can neuroscience assist leadership theorists in better understanding the role of dopamine (interest) and norepinepherine (alertness) in mental performance, and their management through novelty, reward, visualization and other tools?" — Ringleb, A. H. and D. Rock (2008). "The emerging field of NeuroLeadership." *NeuroLeadership Journal NeuroLeadership Institute* info@neuroleadership.org (One): [Full Text] www.NeuroLeadership.org.

≈≈≈≈≈≈≈

Part 4: Two Points: One Hand Here, One Hand There

The touch of your hands can help to heal you much in the same way you can benefit from a soothing massage or treatment from an osteopathic manual therapist, craniosacral therapist or a hands-on physical therapist. The touch of your hands can help you feel and function better even if you don't actually touch, in a similar way to a Reiki Master, Touch for Health nurse or Matrix Energetics practitioner.

To start sit or lie quietly and place one hand on (pick any place) and the other hand on the (pick another place). This is called the *One Hand Here, One Hand There* approach to healing. Following theses exercises is some of the research supporting the idea of touch as a healing modality as well as specific points that may be beneficial to you. You don't have to read or even believe in touch to benefit from it. You only have to try it.

These exercises can be done when you first wake up in the morning. If you hit the snooze button you can keep track of how long it has been. You can do the exercises as a passenger on a long car ride, or before you go to sleep at night. Treating yourself before you go to bed at night will help ensure a more restful sleep.

You never want to judge yourself on what you find (feelings and memories). Know that the feelings that surface are usually from the past. It is almost always something from when you were a child that is surfacing and released.

≈≈≈≈≈≈≈

Exercise: One Hand Here, One Hand There Healing the Body and Brain

This exercise has ten steps, include as many as you can in your practice.

1. This exercise involves placing one hand on one place and the other hand on another place for two minutes or more. A list of locations and why you might want to use them will follow.

You can start by putting one hand on the back of your head where the substantia nigra sits next to the red nucleus in the midbrain at the top of the brain stem. Place the other hand on your heart, slightly to the left of center on your rib cage. With your mind connect the blood flow in your body to your brainstem bringing oxygen and nutrients and drawing away anything you no longer need. Connect your brain and nervous system with the heart, the muscles in the blood vessel walls, visualizing the nervous system flow that runs to the circulatory system supporting the pumping and movement of nourishing blood. You could also think about something relaxing, peaceful or calming.

2. Rest quietly in a sitting or laying down position. Survey the room or space around you and notice your comfort level. What is the most comfortable part of your body?

3. Place one hand on one of the places listed below. There is no need to press, simply be with the area. Notice what you feel.

What is the texture of your clothing or skin? How is the temperature of the area or of your hand? Do you notice a pulsing or buzzing sensation? As Richard Bartlett, developer of Matrix Energetics would say, "Just notice what you notice."

4. Choose a second location for your other hand and notice the ways in which it feel different from where the first hand continues to rest. Are your hands on different colors of clothing, different textures, or different temperatures? How is point A different from point B?

5. While your hands remain on each of their places, again notice the space around you. What colors do you notice? How much light is there in the room? What sounds do you hear? Are there any smells or scents?

6. After a couple of minutes bring your attention back to your hands. What has changed? What new awareness do you have of the texture, temperature, shape, rhythmical movement, color, etc?

7. After five to twenty minutes, when you are ready, get up and notice how your body feels different. What feels better? More flexible? More comfortable?

8. Make some notes about your experience or call someone and share your experience.

9. Drink plenty of water to keep the new flow and experience moving.

10. Repeat this process with the same points or different points as often as you like.

≈≈≈≈≈≈≈

Exercise: One Hand Here, One Hand There Healing with Brain Emotions and Colors

1. This exercise involves placing one hand on one place and the other hand on another place for two minutes or more. A list of locations and why you might want to use them will follow.

To start with place one hand on the back of your head and the other over your lower left rib cage. This hand now covers the liver and gallbladder.

2. Rest quietly in a sitting or laying down position. Survey the room or space around you and notice your

comfort level. What is the most comfortable part of your body?

3. When you have completed a few minutes connecting the head and the liver you can move on to another place. Place one hand on one of the places listed below. There is no need to press, simply be with the area. Notice what you feel.

What is the texture of your clothing or skin? How is the temperature of the area or of your hand? Do you notice a pulsing or buzzing sensation? Just notice what you notice.

4. Choose a second location for your other hand and notice the ways in which it feel different from where the first hand continues to rest. Are your hands on different colors, different textures, or different temperatures? How is point A different from point B?

5. While your hands remain on each of their places, notice the space around you. Is there a feeling you associate with the space? Do you think of that feeling as being positive or negative? What draws your attention when you ask yourself the question, "What emotions do I want to feel? What feelings do I want more of? How do I reach out for more positive feelings in my life?" Just notice what comes up.

6. Close your eyes and visualize each hand as they rest on the chosen locations. What is the color under each hand? Do you see that as a positive or negative color? What comes up as you change with your mind the color to something you feel more comfortable with?

7. After a couple of minutes bring your attention back to your hands. What has changed? What new awareness do you have of the feelings, texture, temperature, shape, rhythmical movement, color, etc?

8. When you are ready get up and notice how your body feels different. What feels better? More flexible? More comfortable?

9. Make some notes about your experience or call someone and share your experience.

10. Drink plenty of water to keep the new flow and experience moving.

11. Feel free to repeat this process as often as you want.

≈≈≈≈≈≈≈

Exercise: One Hand Here, One Hand There Time Travel and Integrating the Past and the Future

1. This exercise involves placing one hand on one place and the other hand on another place for two minutes or more. A list of locations and why you might want to use them will follow.

To start you can put one hand on the back of your head and the other hand on your pelvis, near your hips, digestive system and creative pelvic chakra.

2. Rest quietly in a sitting or laying down position. Survey the room or space around you and notice your comfort level. What is the most comfortable part of your body?

3. Place one hand on one of the places listed below. There is no need to press, simply be with the area. Notice what you feel.

What is the texture of your clothing or skin? How is the temperature of the area or of your hand? Do you notice a pulsing or buzzing sensation? Just notice what you notice.

4. Choose a second location for your other hand and notice the ways in which it feel different from where the first hand continues to rest. Are your hands on different colors, different textures, or different temperatures? How is point A different from point B?

5. While your hands remain on each of their places, look for a number in the space around you, in your mind's eye, or mind's ear (do you hear the sound of a number?). OR focus on a particular age in your past or future.

Do you think of that number or age as being positive or negative? What draws your attention when you ask yourself the question - How old am I in this experience? What is the best thing about the age or experience? What do you want to bring forward from the past or back from the future that can help you in the now? Just notice what comes up.

6. Close your eyes and visualize each hand as they rest on the chosen location. What is the number is under each hand? How does the number feel? What comes up as you change the number to something you feel more comfortable with? Is the number closer or farther from your current age?

Sometimes simply asking yourself the questions will change something and you will be more comfortable and productive.

7. After a couple of minutes bring your attention back to your hands. What has changed? What new awareness do you have of the number, feelings, texture, temperature, shape, rhythmical movement, color, etc?

8. When you are ready get up and notice how your body feels different. What feels better? More flexible? More comfortable?

9. Make some notes about your experience or call someone and share your experience.

10. Drink plenty of water to keep the new flow and experience moving.

11. Feel free to repeat this exercise as many times as you want for as many ages in the past or future as you want.

≈≈≈≈≈≈≈

List of Contact Points, Visualizations and Associated Structures to Use for Brain Health in Parkinson's Disease

Substantia Nigra—the place in the brain that produces dopamine is accessed energetically at the back of the head where the substantia nigra (literally the black stuff) sits next to the red nucleus in the midbrain, which sits like a little elf hat on the top of the brainstem above the pons and medulla of the brainstem. It sits below the sensory thalamus and slightly above and behind the rhythmical and balancing hypothalamus. (More about this later with the Brainstem).

Gallbladder—located behind the lower right side of rib cage, behind and slightly below the liver.

Liver—located behind the lower right side of rib cage.

Limbic system—deep in the brain where the forehead meets the nose and the eyes. The limbic system is a series of nerve fibers that connect the hypothalamus (balance and circadian rhythms) with other areas of the frontal and temporal lobes. The limbic system works by influencing the endocrine (hormonal) system and autonomic nervous system (automatic part of the nervous system - fight / flight and rest / digest). It is a very primitive system and controls the experience and expression of emotions in the body. It allows you to behave in ways that help you express and survive both physical and psychological experience.

The limbic system is associated with
—poor choices
—muscle dysfunctions
—chronic pain
—involuntary movement
—the occurrence of synaesthesia
—creativity
—limbic rage.

Structures in the limbic system include:

a. Amygdala which is involved with
—signaling the cortex (higher brain) about specific stimuli
—critical emotions (disgust and indignation)
—subjective feelings (to remember proper emotional response to a given stimuli)
—eliptoidal personality (shallow mental life, egocentrism aggressiveness, affect occurrence)
—fear and loathing
—vigilance (as well as emotion if expect to have problems)
—unusual shyness
—a high amount of enkephalins (makes you feel good)

Memory dysfunctions are associated with the hippocampus (formation of new declarative or episodic memories), basal ganglia, amygdala (perhaps mediated by through the connections with the hippocampus or with the dorsomedial nucleus of the thalamus (emotional memory) and memory retention and memory loss disorders) septum pellucidum, (willful loss for survival and affected by the limbic region).

The **amygdala** is affected by
—electrocutions
—radiation
—low threshold for electrical discharges
—dysfunctions of vegetative responses, including licking, chewing and seizures

b. Hippocampus is involved with
—the formation of long term memories
—formation of new declarative or episodic memories
—learning if an event is good or bad is associated with the amygdala, while the hippocampus helps to remember event

c. Parahippocampal gyrus is associated with
—spatial memory or remembering where you are in space

d. Cingulate gyrus is associated with

—autonomic functions including heart rate, blood pressure and cognitive processing
—lack of clarity of thought
—confusion
—limbic behaviors
—obsessive compulsive behaviors
—autism
—the placebo effect
—depression

The anterior medial cingulate is a core neural network underlying empathy for pain as well as mindfulness (meditation, visualization) training appears to enhance focused attention in the cingulate gyrus.

The **anterior cingulate gyrus** is also associated with
—happy and pleasant feelings
—self-criticism and with activity
—self-critical thinking to error processing (dorsal anterior cingulate (dAC)
—resolution (dAC)
—behavioral inhibition (dAC)
—emotional tuning (pregenual cingulate)
—activated by painful stimuli (mid-anterior cingulate)
—activated by feelings of guilt for acting counter to social values (subgenual cingulate cortex (SCC)
—altruistic donations towards societal causes (SCC)
—clinical depression (SCC)

Compassionate meditation activates from the left medial prefrontal cortex extending to the anterior cingulate gyrus. The mid-anterior cingulate and premotor cortex have a similar pattern of activation when participants are asked to imagine another's pain from a somatosensory perspective (ie while looking at body parts in painful situations). The areas of the thalamus and the cingulate gyrus become hyperactive in acute schizophrenic patients are important brain areas for perception and communication.

e. Fornix carries signals from the hippocampus to mammillary bodies

f. Hypothalamus regulates the autonomic nervous system via hormone production and release.

Hypothalamus is energetically accessed from each side of the head or from the top of the head.

The hypothalamus is located below the thalamus just above the brain stem and is about the size of an almond. The hypothalamus sends signals to the pituitary gland to stimulate or inhibit hormones which are involved in regulating blood pressure, circadian rhythms (jet lag and sleep disorgers), immune response and body temperature. The hypothalamus responds to many different signals and is connected to many parts of the central nervous system.

The **hypothalamus** is involved with
—regulating blood pressure
—heart rate
—thirst and food intake
—sleep/wake cycle
—others involuntary body functions
—imbalances of water balance
—temperature regulation
—pain, reflex sympathetic dystrophy (basal banglia and substantia nigra and hypothalamus)
—movement disorders
—compassion meditation
—parasympathetic and sympathetic imbalances
—endocrine and pituitary dysfunction
—lack of homeostasis

g. Thalamus helps move signals between the limbic system and the cerebral cortex. The thalamus is a paired structure in the brain situated between the cerebral cortex and the midbrain.

Its function includes
—sending sense and motor signals to the cerebral cortex
—playing a role in the regulation of sleep / wake cycles
—auditory, visual, somatic and visceral functions

Mostly the thalamus has been considered a sort of relay station the only forwards sensory signals. Recently, research suggests that its function is more selective.

The thalamus is associated with
—persistent spontaneous pain
—central pain on the opposite hemibody
—memory dysfunctions
—egocentric
—analgesic or purely algesic thalamic syndrome characterized by contralateral anesthesia (or hypoesthesia), pain disorders, contralateral weakness, somatosensory disturbances, ataxia.

The areas of the thalamus and the cingulate which become hyperactive in acute schizophrenic patients are important brain areas for perception and communication.

h. The mammillary bodies are associated with
—visual impairment
—floaters in the eye
—visual hallucinations
—neuroaggressive behavior
—survival mode
—rage
—neuroaggressive behaviors and rage
—Wilson's Disease

—Thiamine (B1) deficiency affects the mammillary bodies, Wernicke's encephalopathy disease, small petechial bleeds due to alcohol ingestion

Limbic system is a "primitive" emotional circuit. The limbic pathways include the limbic fornix, cingulum, medial forebrain bundle, stria medullaris thalami, olfactory tracts and stria, mammillothalamic tract, stria terminalis, thalamocortical fibers, ventral amygdalofugal path.

Limbic system affective behaviors include
—rage responses
—primitive emotional circuits
—poor judgment
—movement disorders
—chronic pain
—muscle dysfunctions and particularly large muscles.

Note: All of these structures can be energetically accessed by putting one hand over the forehead and eyes.

If you want to support any of these structures and functions, rest one hand on the forehead and eyes and the other hand on the heart or other organ or brain structure.

Basal Ganglia is accessed from the side of the head or top of the center of the head.

The basal ganglia is a group of nuclei located at the base of the forebrain and closely connected to the cerebral cortex and thalamus among others. The basal ganglia is associated with numerous functions including motor control and learning.

The basal ganglia nuclei play a key role in some neurological conditions including some movement disorders and musculoskeletal problems. In addition the basal ganglia dysfunction is involved in Parkinson's disease which is due to the degeneration of dopamine producing cells in the substantia nigra and Huntington's disease, which involves damage to the striatum.

Basal ganglia is associated with
—learning dysfunctions
—Lewy Body disorders (protein folding/fascial strands)
—autonomic nervous system disorders
—extra pyramidal motor system
—somatomotor dysfunctions
—irritable bowel syndrome
—hypervigilance
—anxiety
—reflex sympathetic dystrophy (RSD): basal ganglia, substantia nigra, hypothalamus
—chronic pain

—emotional, motivational, associative and cognitive dysfunctions
—Progressive supranuclear palsy
—neuroendocrine dysfunctions
—Parkinson's disease
—Huntington's Chorea
—dementia (protein folding disorders/fascial strands/Lewy Bodies)
—diabetes (related to inflammation)

Memory dysfunctions including emotional memory (perhaps mediated by through the connections with
—the hippocampus or with the dorsomedial nucleus of the thalamus (memory retention and memory loss disorders)
—septum pellucidum (willful loss for survival)
—Alzheimer's, addictions (also make bad choices)
—sadness and sad memories

Behaviors relative to reward and punishment integration with certain cognitive aspect of the situation as well as the emotional component are associated with the basal ganglia. Emotional imbalances are associated with the basal ganglia and the medial geniculate bodies. Compassion meditation activates the right caudate body extending to the right insula. In contrast, the implicit system is associated with the skill-based knowledge supported primarily by the basal ganglia and has the advantage of being more efficient.

The main components of the basal ganglia include:

a. Striatum

b. Pallidum Globus The pallidus is associated with progressive supranuclear palsy and Parkinson's disease.

c. Subthlamic nucleus

d. Lentiform nucleus associated with osteoporosis, osteopenia, osteomalacia

e. Putamen of the basal ganglia is associated with the
—brain regions compassion training elicited activity in a neural network
—bone health
—the dopaminergic pathways (putamen, globus pallidus).

f. Substantia nigra is part of the midbrain but closely associated with the basal ganglia. The red nucleus, substantia nigra and superior colliculus are all involved in the integrative aspects of motor control.

The midbrain which includes the substantia nigra and the red nucleus is associated with
—Parkinson's disease (substantia nigra)

—motor neurons and cells growth and development (red nucleus)
—involuntary movement disorders
—pride induction engages the posterior medial cortex, a region that has been associated with self-referent processing

One piece of research found the main effect of a compassionate attitude was observed in the midbrain periaqueductal gray (PAG), a region that is activated during pain and the perception of others' pain, and that has been implicated in parental nurturance behaviors. While compassion induction was associated with activation in the midbrain periaqueductal gray, self-reports of compassion experience were correlated with increased activation in a region near the periaqueductal gray, and in the right inferior frontal gyrus (IFG).

Red nucleus is associated with
—involuntary movement disorders (thru rubrospinal tract)
—cell growth and development syndromes
—the integrative aspects of motor control.

The **substantia nigra** is associated with
—movement disorders
—involuntary and voluntary movement
—coordination

—dopamine production (substantia nigra and adrenal medulla also produces it)

—Tourette's syndrome

—movement disorders

—pigmentation and melatonin disorders

—reflex sympathetic dystrophy (RSD)

—chronic pain (basal ganglia, substantia nigra and hypothalamus)

—Alzheimer's, neurodegenerative

—iron toxicity

—verbal aspontaneity (word loss); decreased ability to start talking

—decreased ability in Parkinson's to start with walking

—Lewy body disorders (protein folding/fascial strands)

—voluntary coordination,

—integrative aspects motor control

—ALS (Amytrophic Lateral Sclerosis)

—mercury toxicity and infections with some heavy metals.

Cerebellum is energetically access at the back of the head. The cerebellum is associated with

—pain, reflex sympathetic dystrophy (basal ganglia and substantia nigra and hypothalamus)

—movement disorders, gait, posture and voluntary movement dysfunctions

—ataxia, coordination of the action of various participating muscle groups

—smooth movements

—intention tremors

—intention

—postural reflexes

—balance disturbance

To summarize your hands or someone else's hands (a parent, a friend, or a practitioner) can connect two places as you visualize the connection. Access the areas that seem to be in most need of support and connection including the parts of the brain, the liver and gallbladder, the heart, etc.

For images of brain structures, dopamine and other Parkinson's related information visit http://www.pinterest.com/KimberlyBurnham/parkinson-s-disease-recovery

≈≈≈≈≈≈≈

Exercise: Sleep Solutions

The hypothalamus deep inside the brain is particular important to sleep. A part of the hypothalamus called the suprachiasmic nucleus is also the internal clock mechanism, also known as the biological clock. Use the One Hand Here, One Hand There exercise to improve sleep. About 20 minutes before you plan to go to sleep, lay down with one hand on the back, top or side of the head. The other hand goes on the heart or liver. Rest in this position for 15-20 minutes. You can fall asleep in this position. You can also do this if you wake up in the night before you are ready to get up.

≈≈≈≈≈≈≈

Right Brain and Left Brain in Parkinson's Solutions

This is what four medical experts say about the connection between the corpus callosum (connects the right and left hemisphere) and Parkinson's disease. The corpus callosum as well as contributing to the communication and connection between the right and left hemispheres, can be improved through listening to and creating music, exercises that involve both sides of the body and more.

The corpus callosum can be energetically accessed by putting one hand on the top of your head.

"In Parkinson's disease (PD) cell loss in the substantia nigra is known to result in motor symptoms; however widespread pathological changes occur and may be associated with non-motor symptoms such as cognitive impairment. The data suggest that the corpus callosum or its cortical connections [right brain and left brain] are associated with cognitive impairment in Parkinson's disease patients." —Wiltshire, K., L. Concha, et al. (2010). "Corpus callosum and cingulum tractography in Parkinson's disease." *Can J Neurol Sci* 37(5): 595-600.

"Over the past decade, deep brain stimulation (DBS) has become an effective treatment option for managing severe Parkinson's disease (PD). However, evidence is accumulating that DBS of target sites like the subthalamic nucleus (STN) can result in unintended cognitive effects that lie beyond motor control. Results raise the possibility that the left and right hemisphere might differ in their vulnerability to tolerate side effects on executive functions of DBS treatment." —Lueken, U., M. Schwarz, et al. (2008). "Impaired performance on the Wisconsin Card Sorting Test under left- when compared to right-sided deep brain stimulation of the subthalamic nucleus in patients with Parkinson's disease." *J Neurol* 255(12): 1940-1948.

"Signs of attentional dysfunction mimicking spatial neglect have been described both in humans with lateralized [affects one side of the body more than the other] Parkinson's Disease (PD) and in animals with MPTP-related hemiparkinsonism. Such deficits have been attributed to dopamine loss in basal ganglia and cortical targets." —Garcia-Larrea, L., E. Brousolle, et al. (1996). "Brain responses to detection of right or left somatic targets are symmetrical in unilateral Parkinson's disease: a case against the concept of "parkinsonian neglect'." *Cortex* 32(4): 679-691.

"Speech preparation was measured during speech motor programming in two randomly ordered speech conditions: speech maintenance and switching. These data suggest that left-hemispheric Deep Brain Stimulation may have differential effects on aspects of speech preparation in Parkinson's disease." —Jones, H. N., D. L. Kendall, et al. (2010). "Speech motor program maintenance, but not switching, is enhanced by left-hemispheric deep brain stimulation in Parkinson's disease." *Int J Speech Lang Pathol* 12(5): 385-398.

≈≈≈≈≈≈≈

Exercise: Strengthening the Right and Left Hemisphere Connections

A simple exercise to activate the connection between the right and left hemispheres of the brain is to move in a way that connections the right and left side of your body.

1. March up and down in place while touching the right knee as it rises with the left hand. Then touch the left knee as it rises with the right hand.

For people who can't walk or march up and down in place this can be modified and done in a seated position. Laying down a caregiver can take the person's right hand and touch it to their left hip. You can also visualize doing this exercise.

2. Learn a new musical instrument or play one that you already know. There is extensive medical evidence that music strengthens the connection between the right and left side of the brain.

≈≈≈≈≈≈≈

Introverts and Extroverts: Are You Becoming More Introverted?

There is also research to indicate differences in brain chemistry and brain structure in people who are introverts and extroverts, one of the classifications in the Myers-Brigg Business Personality Test.

"Rigid and introverted personality type has been suggested as possibly associated with risk of Parkinson's disease. Four articles met most selection criteria and three of them reported significant differences in personality features said to be present before Parkinson's onset and between Parkinson's disease cases and controls. Parkinson's cases were more introverted, cautious, socially alert, and tense than controls. Although the instruments used to characterize personality varied widely across studies, the general descriptions of Parkinson's disease patients included nervous, cautious, rigid, and conventional." —Ishihara, L. and C. Brayne (2006). "What is the evidence for a premorbid parkinsonian personality: a systematic review." *Mov Disord* 21(8): 1066-1072.

"It has been suggested that before development of motor symptoms, Parkinson's disease (PD) patients with idiopathic display a specific cluster of personality traits consisting of increased rigidity, conscientiousness, industriousness, orderliness, and cautiousness. The idea of such a distinctive premorbid personality profile remains controversial. Though not differing from medical controls premorbidly, after developing symptoms, PD patients were described as less extroverted; less exploratory and curious; and less organized, goal directed, and disciplined." Glosser, G., C. Clark, et al. (1995). "A controlled investigation of current and premorbid personality: characteristics of Parkinson's disease patients." *Mov Disord* 10(2): 201-206.

"Recent research demonstrated that background noise relative to silence impaired subjects' performance in a cognitively driven odor discrimination test. Subjects were asked to conduct an odor sensitivity task in the presence of either nonverbal noise (e.g., party sound) or verbal noise (e.g., audio book), or silence. With regard to the odor sensitivity task, a significant interaction emerged between the type of background noise and the degree of extraversion. Specifically, verbal noise relative to silence significantly impaired or improved the performance of the odor sensitivity task in the introvert or extrovert group, respectively; the differential effect of introversion/extraversion was not observed in the nonverbal noise-induced task performance." —Seo, H. S., A. Hahner, et al. (2012). "Influence of background noise on the performance in the odor sensitivity task: effects of noise type and extraversion." *Exp Brain Res* 222(1-2): 89-97.

≈≈≈≈≈≈≈

Exercise: One Hand Here, One Hand There

In addition to the above exercises, the connection between the sides of the brain and the corpus callosum can be improved with the one hand here and one hand there technique. For example, you can place one hand on the top of the head holding each side of the brain and the other hand over the heart or the liver. Or one hand could be on the right side of the head and the other hand on the heart or lungs.

Corpus callosum is energetically access at the top of the head. The corpus callosum connects the right and left sides of the brain and is associated with
—post traumatic stress disorder (PTSD)
—autism
—obsessive compulsive
—verbal aspontaneity
—hypergraphia (always writing)
—Parkinson's and Schizophrenia symptoms.

≈≈≈≈≈≈≈

Right Cortical Hemisphere / Right Side of the Brain

The right side of the cortical or higher brain is associated with

—the negative emotions of sadness, fear, and disgust

—occurrence of synaesthesia

—relation to creativity

—awareness perceived directly

—implicit, intuitive thoughts

—accepts an ever-changing world

—favors subjective experiences that provide direct awareness of the world.

—favors the experienced essence of the world, including all sensory details

—moving, changing, constantly innovating and evolving in new ways

—the world is alive in every aspect of its essence, including the spiritual

—the body is a whole that includes emotional, psychological and spiritual aspects

—metaphors, imagery, myths, music and other creative arts convey experiences that invite direct awareness of the world

—embodied experiences provide knowledge about the world

—'Knowledge' and 'truth' … [is] personal, provisional, a matter of degree, a journey."

—we feel "a desire or *longing* towards something, something that lies beyond itself, towards the other."

—accepting being part of an uncontrollable, ever shifting world

—every element of the world must be respected

—metaphors, imagery, music and other creative arts convey experiences that invite direct awareness of the world

—circular, parallel

—concerned for the good of all

—self-reflective

—is inclusive of LH awareness

≈≈≈≈≈≈≈

Left Brain Dominant

—When given a task or assignment, you don't always need to know why it's important.

—You get a great deal of pleasure in creating to-do lists and checking each item off as it is accomplished.

—You would prefer Sudoku puzzles over getting messy with clay.

—When shopping for a new car, you would probably look at fuel efficiency and crash safety ratings over the looks of the car.

—When traveling, you like to have your itinerary completely planned down to the last detail.

—Because you respond to verbal cues, you prefer lectures to textbooks.

—You are good at remembering names.

—Your office is neatly organized with a place for everything. You spend little time looking for things.

—When trying a new software program, you prefer to use the instruction manual.

—You are almost always on time or early for meetings and appointments.

≈≈≈≈≈≈≈

Left Cortical Hemisphere / Left Side of the Brain

The left side of the cortical or higher brain is associated with

—the positive emotions of happiness and amusement

—awareness built upon bits of chosen and researched information

—explicit

—rational

—favors objectively measurable data

—favors sight and appearances

—static, fixed, inflexible in theoretical orientation

—the world is composed of inert particles

—the body is composed of interacting but inert particles

—words and ideas define facts about the world

—logical constructs about the world, "representation" of the world, is what is real

—'Knowledge' and 'truth' … [is] impersonal, static, complete, a thing

—favors a static worldview

—the world is here to be used to serve human needs

—seeks to control the world

—the world is just a bunch of resources, to be enjoyed and exploited by humanity

—words and ideas define facts about the world

—linear, sequential

—utilitarian in ethic

—over-confident in its understanding of reality, questioning its own views and seeking consensual validations

—lacking insight into its problems

—excludes and dismisses RH awareness

≈≈≈≈≈≈≈

Right Brain Dominant

—When given a task or assignment, you want to know why it's important because you like the big picture.

—You don't need to-do lists because you like to wing it.

—You would prefer modeling clay into pottery over Sudoku puzzles because it is more creative.

—When shopping for a new car, you would probably pick what looks best, rather than what drives best.

—When traveling, you like impulsive adventure: Why plan it all out and ruin it?

—Because you are visual, you prefer textbooks to lectures.

—You can remember a person's face but not necessarily their name.

—Your office is not necessarily organized but you find what you need, eventually.

—When trying a new software program, you install it and immediately begin experimenting with it.

—You aren't always on time, even if you mean to be.

≈≈≈≈≈≈≈

Right Brain Exercise

If you exhibited more right brain dominant traits, you are a global thinker. Try the following when starting a new project:

1. Get organized
2. Work on developing time management skills
3. Use spatial organizers when taking notes
4. Draw diagrams
5. Try visualizing the information presented in your notes
6. Recite information
7. Use mnemonics
8. Use rhythmic activities
9. Use movement
10. Listen to music while exercising (as long as it is not distracting!)

≈≈≈≈≈≈≈

Left Brain Exercise

If you exhibited more left brain dominant traits, you are an analytical thinker. Try the following when starting a new project:

1. Plan a regular schedule
2. Recognize and identify organizational patterns
3. Use memory devices
4. Take precise notes
5. Practice/rehearse information on a routine basis

≈≈≈≈≈≈≈

Exercise: Right and Left Brain One Hand Here

1. Place one hand on one side of your head and the other on one of the organs.
2. Then place one hand on the other side of your head and the other hand on one of the organs.
3. What difference do you notice between one side of your head and the other?
4. Do different emotions or ideas come up when you place a hand on the right side compared to the left side?

≈≈≈≈≈≈≈

Hands-On Emotions

These are the locations and the energetic and emotional ideas behind different areas in your body. These suggestions come from the ancient ideas of acupuncture and acupressure as well as the more recent field of Integrative Manual Therapy and Matrix Energetics.

To use this information in the one hand here, one hand there exercises, simply place one hand in the location of the organ or structure and place the other hand on an area of the head associated with the brain structure you are trying to support. Visualize the connection for five to ten minutes as you relax and feel your body.

≈≈≈≈≈≈≈

Organs and Structures

You can also connect these organs and structures to each other. For example, place one hand on the area of the ureters (either along the lower back or abdomen) and the other hand over the heart for five to ten minutes as you relax and breathe. Notice what changes.

1. **Ureters,** across the low back, 1 inch on either side of spine (at waist level). You can access the ureters with the back or front of your hand and forearm. The Ureters are

the Center for toxic drainage. Take all these Process Centers to the ureters at least once for physical and emotional drainage. The ureters are great for first aid for physical trauma (ie) a sprained ankle; you put one hand over the ureters and the other hand over the ankle. Typically, this will decrease pain and swelling. The ureters are the tubes between the kidneys and the bladder and so are part of the urogenital system. In Traditional Chinese Medicine the kidneys and bladder are considered to be water elements and associated with the color blue. Notice what is blue around you as you connect the ureters to other areas.

2. **Frontals or Forehead**: Thought, Judgment, Behavior. Great for ADD. Specific to Emotional Health focus above the Right eye at the hairline (or where it used to be) for balancing emotional health. For Mental Health focus above Left eye at the hairline to release thoughts or perseveration.

3. **Limbic System** at the bridge of nose or frontonasal and eyes is your center for survival and has to do with the rage responses. Think of a lion that has been attacked and wounded. This is not anger, it is pure rage. There are no rational thoughts associated with rage. Here between the eyes is also the sixth chakra, the third eye which is associated with the color violet. Notice if you have any six-sided objects in your environment.

4. **Parietal lobe** at the top of the head is the home of the sensory and motor cortex and associated with feelings and sensations (sight, sound, taste, smell, and touch) as well as actions and movements. This is also the area of the seventh chakra, the crown chakra, connecting us to the sky and our environment. It is associated with the color purple or white. Meditate on the sky as you connect this area to other places in your body. What color is the sky? What can it tell you about the outside temperature or weather?

5. **Occipital lobe** at the back of the head is the visual cortex associated with vision, visual sensations, and perception. What are you seeing? What do you want to see? How do you feel about what you see right now?

6. **Temporal lobe** is on the right and left side of the head and is connected with hearing, balance, and stability. What are you hearing? What are you saying as every cell in your body listens? Is your life balanced? Is your body balanced? What does balance mean?

7. **Thyroid** in Front of the Neck and Throat Area is about expression or not expressing yourself (verbally, creatively, etc) because of fear or other emotions. This is also the area of the throat chakra associated with the color blue. In Traditional Chinese Medicine the thyroid is often associated with the Triple Warmer meridian and the Pericardium (tough outer protective layer of the

heart). They are fire elements associated with the color red. As you visualize your throat and thyroid and all that passes through this area is it more associated with blue or red or some other color or an emotion?

8. **Heart** (Center of the Chest a little to the Left) is connected to love, joy, hatred, loss of love (ie) abandonment. This is also the area of the heart chakra, associated with the color green. In Traditional Chinese Medicine from which acupuncture and acupressure come, the heart has a meridian or line of energy associated with the small intestine and the color red. Both of these fire element meridians run along the arms through the shoulders, elbows, and hands. Notice the energy flow in your body as you connect the heart with other spots.

9. **Lungs** at the front and back are connected to grief and deep sadness, despair, oxygen and your will to live life. The lung meridian is paired with the large intestines and the color white. These are metal elements. The parts of the large intestine include from the right hip: cecum, ascending colon, transverse colon, descending colon, and at the left hip the sigmoid colon. Notice your breathing and what changes as you connect the lungs to other organs or the head.

10. **Spleen** on the Left side of rib cage, between rib 8 and rib 10: disappointment in mankind (ie) war veteran, or

someone who has experienced terror or abuse could have a lot of emotion locked in the spleen. The spleen, pancreas and stomach are paired in Traditional Chinese Medicine and considered earth elements and associated with the color yellow.

11. **Liver** (Lower Right Rib Cage): anger and detoxification. Liver and gallbladder are paired in Traditional Chinese Medicine along with the color green. Both are wood elements.

12. **Pancreas** just below Center and Left side of rib cage, in the Abdomen: major issues of significance (life or death) consider your path and purpose in this life. "What am I supposed to do in life?" The third chakra or the solar plexus is also in this area and is associated with the color yellow.

13. **Kidneys** lower rib cage at the back. You can use your hand and forearm on the front or back of the low back and abdomen to work with fear, anxiety, depression, and fluid regulation. Blue water elements the kidney and bladder acupuncture meridians run down the legs.

14. **Prostate or Uterus** just above pubic bone in the front of the pelvis: sexuality, gender, reproduction. There are two meridians that circle the center line of the body. In the front the conception vessel and in the back the governing vessel. These can be energetically connected

by touching the tip of your tongue to the gums inside and above the upper teeth.

15. **Upper Arms** (both): Control over self, self control. Are you in control? Who tries or has tried to control you? Are we ever really in control?

These associations regarding the arms were developed by Sharon W Giammatteo in her book, *Body Wisdom*, where there is also more information about the process centers.

16. **Lower Arms** (both): Belief systems. What do you believe? Who do you believe? Do your belief systems serve you?

17. **Cecum** (beginning part of the large intestine or colon) in front of the Right Hip: digestion, absorption, what are you holding on to? It can also be associated with gluten sensitivity and allergies. The first chakra (red) is located in the pelvis and the sacral chakra (orange) is also nearby.

For an image of these locations visit https://www.linkedin.com/today/post/article/2014052916 1725-39038923

≈≈≈≈≈≈≈

Touch Related References

"Abnormal somatosensory processing [somato = body, sensory = sensations, processing = take in the information and understand it] may contribute to motor impairments observed in Parkinson's disease (PD). Dopaminergic medications have been shown to alter somatosensory processing such that tactile perception is improved. In PD, it remains unclear whether the temporal sequencing of tactile stimuli is altered and if dopaminergic medications alter this perception."— Nelson, A. J., A. Premji, et al. (2012). "Dopamine alters tactile perception in Parkinson's disease." *Can J Neurol* Sci 39(1): 52-57.

"Which is heavier: a pound of lead or a pound of feathers? This classic trick question belies a simple but surprising truth: when lifted, the pound of lead feels heavier--a phenomenon known as the size-weight illusion. Our findings suggest that two fundamentally different strategies for the integration of prior expectations with sensory information coexist in the nervous system for weight estimation." —Brayanov, J. B. and M. A. Smith (2010). "Bayesian and "anti-Bayesian" biases in sensory integration for action and perception in the size-weight illusion." *J Neurophysiol* 103(3): 1518-1531.

"The patient's involuntary muscle contractions of the neck were relieved by classical sensory tricks such as touching her cheek and grasping the posterior neck. She also noted an interesting phenomenon that her dystonic movements were reduced with visual maneuvers, such as looking at herself in the mirror." —Lee, C. N., M. Y. Eun, et al. (2012). ""Visual sensory trick" in patient with cervical dystonia." *Neurol Sci* 33(3): 665-667. [Full Text] http://link.springer.com/content/pdf/10.1007%2Fs10072-011-0831-x

What the research is saying about the value of touch, using your own hands or getting a treatment from someone else. Many of these references and quotes are from Medline, which indexes the most reputable journal article in the field of medicine.

Touch or contact with the two areas is all that is needed to make a shift. "The experience of being touched, new research shows, has direct and crucial effects on the growth of the body as well as the mind." — Goleman, D. (1988). "The Experience of Touch: Research Points to a Critical Role." *New York Times February 2.* http://query.nytimes.com/gst/fullpage.html?sec=health&res=940DE0D91F3EF931A35751C0A96E948260.

The *New York Times* article goes on to say, "Touch is a means of communication so critical that its absence retards growth in infants, according to researchers who are for the first time determining the neurochemical effects of skin-to-skin contact. The new work focuses on the importance of touch itself, not merely as part of, say, a parent's loving presence. The findings may help explain the long-noted syndrome in which infants deprived of direct human contact grow slowly and even die."

Hands-on contact can shift brain chemistry, which certainly affects how we feel and function. "New research suggests that certain brain chemicals released by touch, or others released in its absence, may account for these infants' failure to thrive. The studies on the physiology of touch come against a backdrop of continuing research on the psychological benefits of touch for emotional development." —Goleman, D. (1988). "The Experience of Touch: Research Points to a Critical Role." *New York Times February 2.* http://query.nytimes.com/gst/fullpage.html?sec=health&r es=940DE0D91F3EF931A35751C0A96E948260

"The ancient practice of acupressure may be able to calm the aggressive behavior that often results from dementia, a small study suggests. One of the most common symptoms of Alzheimer's disease and other forms of dementia is agitation. It's expressed in any number of ways. Some people with dementia yell at or physically attack other people, while others habitually undress themselves or wander." —Reuters (2007). "Acupressure eases Alzheimer's agitation." *Chinese Medicine News Revolution News theme* by Brian Gardner: {Full   Text] http://chinesemedicinenews.com/2007/2004/2010/acupressure-eases-alzheimers-agitation/.

One study looked at the influence of touch on the ability to feel that area. Researchers explain, "The mature mammalian nervous system alters its functional organization in a use-dependent manner." This means the more you touch an area the better the sensation in that location. Continuing they said, "Enhanced stimulation of a body part enlarges its cortical representational zones and may change its topographic order." —Sterr, A., M. M. Muller, et al. (1998). "Perceptual correlates of changes in cortical representation of fingers in blind multifinger Braille readers." *J Neurosci* 18(11): 4417-4423.

The brain is more tuned into an area that is touched. Researchers concluded that touch can be associated with changes in an individual's sensations and behavior.

≈≈≈≈≈≈≈

Part 5: Applying Social Psychology to the Community of Cells in Your Body

This section is about how we can look at the community of cells that make up the brain, the nervous system and the body and what we can learn from social psychology and business models that focus on community organization, productivity and relationships.

≈≈≈≈≈≈≈

Exercise: The Business of the Brain and Visual Acuity: Do You Have Questions?

There are some interesting organizational dynamics based on our brain and nervous system function that are currently being applied by David Rock and his coaching staff to work environments and businesses. It can also be applied with positive outcomes to your physical health and eyesight.

David Rock has written several fascinating books on how our brains either supports us to think clearly and have insights or work against our decision making process. He has developed the field of *Neuroleadership*, an emerging field of study focused on bringing neuroscientific knowledge into the areas of leadership development, management training, change management, education, consulting and coaching.

While David Rock doesn't apply his work to physical health. Many of his ideas on interpersonal relationships and productivity can be applied to the community of cells that contribute to your health. For example, David Rock's SCARF model involves five domains of human social experience: Status, Certainty, Autonomy, Relatedness & Respect, and Fairness.

Think about an area of your body, which you wish functioned better, was more productive, more efficient, or which supported you to be better able to accomplish your purpose in life.

Now consider these questions. You don't need to find all the answers completely for this exercise to have benefit. Just asking the question can have a positive impact because it directs your attention to the areas and this through biofeedback mechanisms can improve blood flow and nervous system connection to the area. You can also put one of your hands on the area to further draw your attention to it.

Exercise: Fill in the blank........

What is the status of _____ in my body as a whole? What can be done to increase the status or how that area feels?

For example, what is the status of the liver in my body? Consider for a moment what is status in a physical sense. Someone with higher status often has more resources available. So consider what does the liver need in terms of resources. One thing is blood flow carrying nutrient, especially proteins. So eating better quality protein can increase the status of the liver. Also in Traditional Chinese Medicine, the liver is associated with anger issues. So finding ways to address anger in productive ways increases the status of the liver. Both of these things also increase over all health in the body. In acupuncture the liver meridian, an energetic flow of information, is associated with the eyes and eye health. Is your vision for your business and life being filtered through an angry liver or one with high status?

How does certainty or uncertainty in my life affect _____?

For example, how does certainty in my life affect my knees? One way to increase certainty for your knees is to always walk on even, level surfaces. That way your knees and legs can be more certain about how they should move and balance. A surprise, an unexpected curb or crack in the sidewalk can throw your balance off and cause a fall. On the other hand a life with no variability is well ... boring. A different way to increase certainty is to increase the amount of incoming information on which our balance is predicated.

If my eyes are good and I can see the curb, then my knees will know how to deal with it, how to adapts or adjust so that my walking is smooth. Wearing shoes that are comfortable and also allow for more information to travel from the point of contact with the ground up to my brain and balance centers also allows me to adjust appropriately as I walk into a hotel ballroom to talk about the importance of vision.

Can _____ do its job in my body in an autonomous way and is it properly supported?

For example, Can the lungs do their job in an autonomous way? Obviously, the lungs are surrounded by the rib cage and the neck and shoulder above and the diaphragm below. Compression from any of these areas makes it harder for the lungs to do their job. Also if the liver is adhered (due to trauma or inflammation) to the diaphragm, then every time the diaphragm contracts and relaxes it has to drag the liver along for the ride. Hands-on Myofascial Release by a massage therapists or physical therapist to release restrictions can ensure the autonomy of the lungs. Breathing exercises can also help support lung function as can dealing with the emotions of grief and sadness, often associated in acupuncture with the lungs.

How is _____ related to its neighbors, blood flow in the body, or nutrient flow through the physical self?

For example, how is the sacrum related to its neighbors, which include the lumbar spine, hips, colon, uterus / prostate, bladder, etc? Our center of gravity is at the sacrum. It is also the end of the digestive system and the renal (kidney & bladder) system and intimately involved with our reproductive system. The sacrum is the interface between the spine and the legs and between the right and left side of the body. Consider how exercise, eating with intention, or healthy sexual relationships can improve the relationship of the sacrum to the surrounding areas. In an energy medicine approach using chakras, the sacral area is also an area of creativity, of physically manifesting a brain generated ideas into reality.

Entrepreneurial expert, Brendon Burchard and psychiatrist, Daniel Amen talk about using the mind to heal the brain. Neuroscience research connects the frontal lobe (your cognitive and voluntary movement centers) with creativity and caring. These three can form a triangle of influence. Improving your creativity stimulates cognitive function and your ability to care about the world around you. Doing things to improve your cognitive ability also contributes to a more creative and caring expression.

How do I show respect for _____? Is it fair how this area is treated?

For example, how do I show respect for my heart? Dietary and exercise choices certainly influence how fairly or respectfully the heart is being treated. Doing the things you feel passionate about, the things that call to you and bring you joy (the emotion most associated with the heart) also influence heart health and how each cell in the heart interacts with each other heart cell and with the whole community of cells that make up your body.

Think about an area of your body, which you wish functioned better. Now consider these questions. You don't need to find all the answers completely for this exercise to have benefit. Just asking the question can have a positive impact because it directs your attention to the areas and through biofeedback mechanisms can improve blood flow and nervous system connection to the area. You can also put one of your hands on the area to further connect with it and draw your attention to it. You can choose to fill in the blank with the eyes, as in what is the status of the eyes? Or with an area of your body experiencing pain or symptoms. Or you can apply this model to your employees and business.

1. What is the status of _____ in my body as a whole? What can be done to increase the status or how that area feels?

2. How does certainty or uncertainty in my life affect ___?

3. Can _____ do its job in my body in an autonomous way and is it properly supported?

4. How _____ is related to its surrounding neighbors, blood flow in the body, or nutrient flow in the body?

5. How do I show respect for _____ of my body? Is it fair how this area is treated?

≈≈≈≈≈≈≈

More information on the SCARF model can be found at www.your-brain-at-work.com/files/NLJ_SCARFUS.pdf

≈≈≈≈≈≈≈

Part 6: Acupressure's Gallbladder Meridian Points and the Homunculus or Little Man in the Brain

Taping the side of your eye can stimulate dopamine balance in the body. In acupuncture the gallbladder meridian points GB 1 and GB 3 are found at the side of the eye. As I work with clients with a range of neurological disorders including, Parkinson's disease, multiple sclerosis, Huntington's disease, autism, macular degeneration and Alzheimer's disease, I have found that certain acupressure meridians are associated with certain neurotransmitters or brain chemicals. The gallbladder meridian is associated with dopamine levels in the body. Along the gallbladder meridian the easiest to access reflex points are along the outer leg and over the ears on each side of the head. The gallbladder meridian connects the head to the toes.

The idea of lightly tapping on points on the body comes from many fields of complementary and alternative medicine including Emotional Freedom Technique (EFT), where practitioners guide you through a series of points as you hold new thoughts in your mind and say affirmations. The goal is to integrate a new consciousness of your power and creativity into your consciousness, subconscious and body awareness.

Imagine the top of the brain with a homunculus [little human form], like the body of a little person inside the brain draped along the top of the head. Because we get the most sensation from our hands and lips, the representation of the hands and lips are larger, out of proportion to the rest of the body of the homunculus.

The homunculus is a slice through the brain with the nerves that supply and get feedback from your physical arms, legs, skin, trunk, lips, hands, etc.

Now imagine that there are acupuncture meridians running through your physical body as well as the representation of the physical body in the brain. Those brain arms, legs, face and body of the homunculus are little bunches of neurons in the brain carrying, feelings, sending out the energy that flows through your meridian system.

Visualize a tiny fractal-like liver in the brain, a reflection and communication center for the physical liver, the emotion of anger and compassion that flows through the liver meridian up and down the legs. Each liver meridian point surrounded by nerve endings communicating between the legs and the brain. Red hot anger or light pink compassion welling up from each liver meridian point, the liver under the rib cage on the right side as well as the liver of the brain's homunculus. All connected—all flowing, releasing, sharing, expressing your inner self.

≈≈≈≈≈≈

Harnessing the Circadian Chinese Clock for Deeper Sleep, Better Vision, and Brain Health

In Traditional Chinese Medicine and acupuncture there is a rhythm or flow of energy through a system of meridians, lines of vibration with reflex points along the way. Each meridian or organ system holds the energy at the highest level for two hours in a 24 hour day. Then the energy flows into the next meridian, supporting healing and function as it moves.

There are lots of ways to use this information to improve your circadian sleep rhythms for deeper sleep, as well as better brain focus, attention, vision, hearing, and sensation.

For example Liver congestion can cause headaches, restlessness and insomnia. The liver is most active from 1 am to 3 am. If you wake up between these times, one way to get back to sleep is to put one hand over the liver in the lower right hand side of the rib cage and the other hand over your head or your heart. Connecting the two areas for a few minutes can have a calming and relaxing effect on the liver allowing for better energy flow and sleep to return. You can also visualize a color, shape or feeling along the organ and its meridian that can improve the blood flow to the organ and increase your overall health. For the liver that color could be the green associated with the Wood elements in Traditional Chinese Medicine (Liver and gallbladder).

The gallbladder is the other wood element and is associated with the color green and the neurotransmitter dopamine. While acetylcholine (the neurotransmitter of connections—of nerve connections) is associated with the stomach meridian, the color yellow and the earth element.

≈≈≈≈≈≈≈

Here are the names of the acupuncture organ meridian and the times they are considered to be most active.

The Wood Elements for Growth & Vitality: **Gallbladder** 11 pm–1 am and **Liver** 1–3 am; green color, anger emotion, compassion virtue.

The Metal Elements for Clarity & Precision: **Lung** 3–5 am; **Large Intestine** 5–7 am; white color, grief emotion, justice virtue.

The Earth Elements for Nourishment & Stability: **Stomach** 7–9 am; **Spleen / Pancreas** 9–11am; yellow color, worry and disappointment emotion, faith virtue.

The Fire Elements for Passion & High Energy: **Heart** 11 am–1 pm; **Small Intestine** 1–3 pm; red color, joy / mania emotion, propriety and courtesy virtue.

The Water Elements for Ease & Abundance: **Bladder** 3–5 pm; **Kidney** 5–7 pm; blue color, fear emotion, wisdom virtue.

Two more Fire Elements: **Pericardium** 7–9 pm; **Triple Warmer** (endocrine and temperature regulation) 9–11 pm; red color, joy / mania emotion, propriety and courtesy virtue.

Let's say you wanted more abundance in your life. Between 3 pm and 7 pm during the water element's period you could do a visualization around flow through the bladder and kidneys or imagine energy warming the bladder and kidneys or do a stretch for the mid back area (around the kidneys) and pelvic area (bladder) to free up and relax this area.

For improvements in your digestive system consider what you are eating during the times when the small intestine (site of most absorption of food) is most active. For better circulation consider what you are eating for lunch while the heart is most active.

You can also stimulate these points in other ways, including acupressure (pressing and rubbing) and using an Integrative Manual Therapy clicker or a chiropractic speeder board, kinesio-elastic tape on the point, tuning forks or even your voice to mechanically and energetically vibrate the points. These points can be stimulated by colored light, by the colors you wear over the point, by a drop of aromatherapy, homeopathic solutions, Bach flower remedies or Reiki symbols on the point.

In reflexology your finger tips are reflective of the sinuses, so tapping or rubbing using your finger tips can stimulate better drainage from the sinuses, enhance breathing and oxygenation of the brain and the body. In acupuncture the finger tips stimulate the various meridians including the six arm meridians: heart, small intestine, lung, large intestine, pericardium and triple warmer.

≋≋≋≋≋≋≋

Emotional Freedom Technique Tapping and Brain Chemistry

For an example of how tapping can influence brain chemistry let's look at the side of the eye or the bony border outside the corner of the eye, which is a point used in Emotional Freedom Technique's (EFT) tapping. In acupuncture this area includes the Tai yang extra point, and the gallbladder meridian points GB 1 and GB 3. It is also a place of intersection where four cranial bones meet: the frontal bone, temporal bone, parietal bone and the sphenoid. It is the intersection point of the Gallbladder, Triple Warmer and Stomach Meridians. These intersection points are associated with the temporal [time] bone, the TMJ or jaw, and the temporal lobe, which is the seat of your hearing, balance and a sense of time [past, present, future].

The gallbladder meridian which runs along the eye as well as down the legs is associated with the brain chemical or neurotransmitter, dopamine. Balanced dopamine leads to strong comfortable movement, a sense of reality and creativity, as well as a view of the things that are rewarding in your life and the ability to see the opportunities in the present and imagine them in the future. GB 1 is also associated with good decision making abilities, inspiration behind decisions and when out of balance leads to irritability, rage, bitterness, constant sadness, as well as anger of the sort that leads to irrational or hasty decisions and allergies.

One study showed that acupuncture as well as stroking of the skin changed neurotransmitter balances, improving nervous system function, alertness, blood pressure and bladder control. Researchers said, "There are significant age-related changes in autonomic nervous system function that are responsible for an impaired ability to adapt to environmental or intrinsic visceral stimuli in the elderly. We review data on changes in autonomic nervous system regulation of cardiovascular and urinary function, as well as data on strategies to improve function. There is data showing alterations in peripheral and central autonomic nerve activity, and decreases in neurotransmitter receptor action that lead to diminished autonomic reactivity (e.g. blood pressure and cerebral blood flow regulation) and poorly coordinated autonomic discharge (e.g. bladder function). Simple strategies for autonomic function improvement and increasing cortical blood flow include walking and somatic afferent stimulation (ie stroking the skin or receiving acupuncture) to increase sympathetic, parasympathetic and central cholinergic activity." — Hotta, H. and S. Uchida (2010). "Aging of the autonomic nervous system and possible improvements in autonomic activity using somatic afferent stimulation." *Geriatr Gerontol Int* 10 Suppl 1: S127-136.

≈≈≈≈≈≈≈

Exercise: Tapping on Acupuncture Points

1. Start by tapping five times gently on the side of the eye and above and below the eyes.

2. Notice how your hand feels and how the point feels. Does the point feel flexible, strong, and/or warm? How would you describe the texture of the skin and the tissue below the skin?

3. Tap each point five times, then stop and look inside. What does the point feel like? What is changed by your tapping?

4. Notice whether you want to keep tapping or if that is enough.

5. Is there a color, a number, shape or emotion that you associate with this point.

Variations:

Once you are finished tapping look around your space. What has changed? Are the colors more vibrant? Has the temperature changed? Then notice what has changed in your body. Get up and feel what has changed in your movement or walking.

As an additional exercise you can wear different colors of clothing or hat over a point and walk around noticing whether your movement is better with one color or another.

Or you can put a drop of the Bach Flower Remedy - Rescue Remedy or Heel's Homeopathic Remedy - Traumeel on the point and then move around and notice what improves.

Points Along the Liver Meridian

The liver meridian is associated with norepinephrine balance in the body.

This is what researchers had to say about acupuncture points and neurotransmitters. "After treatment [acupuncture], Dopamine content increased significantly in the acupuncture group with a significant difference as compared with that of the control group; and after treatment Norepinephrine and 5-hydroxy-indoleacetic acid (5-HIAA) contents in the two groups significantly increased as compared with that before treatment. Acupuncture can benignly [without harm] and comprehensively regulate general functions, and increase contents of monoamines [dopamine, noradrenaline, adrenaline and serotonin] in the body, so as to play the role of anti-depression." —Zhou, S. H. and F. D. Wu (2007). "[Therapeutic effect of acupuncture on female's climacteric depression and its effects on DA, NE and 5-HIAA contents]." *Zhongguo Zhen Jiu* 27(5): 317-321.

≈≈≈≈≈≈≈

Part 7: Flow Along Fractal Pathways and Vision Exercises

Would your walking and movement improve if you could see more clearly, if you could take in information about your environment, for example, the texture of the walkway, the tilt of the slope, the traction of your shoes?

This section includes a fractal vision exercise to increase your perception of all that is around you as well as the opportunities and resources available to you.

"French mathematician Benoit Mandelbrot coined a single word to describe a wide range of geometric structures or patterns found throughout nature, including trees, coastlines, our own branching blood vessel tree, the layers of tissue in the small intestines, and the neural network of our brain. The term is "fractals," and it describes the richly-textured self-similar shapes existing everywhere. A tree is an example of a fractal.

Each branch resembles a smaller version of the trunk. Even the leaves have tiny, branching veins which are self-similar to the branching trunk. A tree is visually complex, but it is made up of one simple branching pattern. The self-similar structures, patterns, processes, and information inside and outside your body share similarities with nature. You are an integral part of the pattern that forms the natural world—held by it, included within it, and safe to explore the opportunities it provides for learning and growth.

You can become healthier by simply appreciating or observing the beauty of natural scenes and by recognizing the fractal patterns they contain. People recover from major surgery far more quickly when placed in hospital rooms with windows looking out on natural scenery. By looking for and recognizing patterns, you can easily create your own stress-reducing exercises and see how you fit into the whole.

Which patterns and images make you healthier? Where is your community? What are you contributing to it and to your own life?

Your brain--that intersection between mind, body, and spirit--contains nerves branching like the limbs of a tree, and due to this fractal design, you can communicate with others and perceive the world around and inside yourself. A healthy brain can process information in a way that "fits" a personal landscape shaped by attitudes, previous knowledge, and experience. Each time you encounter something new, you change the contours of your nervous system; you change "the fit." Each time you notice something different, you extend the life of your healthy brain.

Do you notice differences or changes each time you reevaluate and reinterpret the experiences in your life?" —An Excerpt from Kimberly Burnham, PhD, The Nerve Whisperer (2011) "*Our Fractal Nature, a Journey of*

Self-Discovery and Connection." $6.95 ISBN: 978-1-937207-01-4

www.amazon.com/Kimberly-Burnham/e/B0054RZ4A0

"Become empowered by your fractal nature! *Our Fractal Nature* guides you through concepts and fun exercises to shape your personal healing potential to fit your needs. Tap into fractals to find new energy resources and expand self-awareness. Learn to recognize fractal patterns in your life, select the seed for each beginning, and surf life's rhythms so you can choose to live in a friendly universe!"

≈≈≈≈≈≈≈

Exercise: The Fractal Patterns of the Diversity Tree

Just noticing the pattern, the way in which we are similar and are connected can bring healing, strengthen the function of your brain, and help you to be more adaptable. This all makes breakfast more fun in the morning.

Many of the patterns in the natural world are fractal in nature. Fractals are a mathematical description of a rough, uneven shape. An oak tree has a fractal shape with a self similar branching pattern. One of the characteristics of fractal patterns that the big thing is like the small thing only bigger. A tree for example has a trunk with branches. Each branch with its own branches is like the trunk only smaller. Even tiny leaves have a trunk like vein which shows a branching pattern. The vein in the leaf is like the tree trunk only much, much smaller.

Often your eyes relax when you notice this natural pattern and the similarity of shapes, whether it is a bright red maple tree in the fall or a tall blue spruce or an oak tree seedling. And when we are relaxed, our blood flows through our fractal branching blood vessels bringing nourishing oxygen and nutrients to our fractal patterned brain. There is scientific research that suggests we heal faster, with less pain in a hospital room with window that looks out over a natural scene with fractal shaped popular trees, red tulips, blades of blue green grass with fractal shaped mountain ranges, puffy white clouds or a jagged shoreline in the distance.

Try this Fractal Tree Vision exercise outside in a place that has trees, when you have a chance. Or you can at each step close your eyes and do this as a visualization, imagining a huge beautiful tree. The healing properties of noticing the natural patterns seems to work even when you are looking at a painting of a tree or natural landscape.

1. Look around yourself. Notice the light. How bright is it? Notice the colors and shapes around you. This is the "before" measurement of how you feel in your skin and in your environment. Notice how you feel, how relaxed

your head and shoulders are. Feel whether every part of your body is comfortable. Take a minute or two to check in with your body and emotions. Then take a minute or two with each of these steps.

2. Choose a tree for this exercises (real or imagined or a painting). Stand about 20 feet or seven meters from the tree. Notice the overall shape. Do you recognize the kind of tree it is? It doesn't matter if you do. Are there any birds that you see or hear? Are there any crickets or bugs making sounds? Is there a wind blowing, moving the tree? Notice the overall color of the leaves and branches.

3. Walk a little closer, so that you are about 10 feet or three meters from the tree. What is different from this distance? Do you notice more detail in the roughness of the bark? Notice the angle at which the branches come off the central trunk. See how the leaves are not all the same color and that there are shades and variation in the leaves. Does your body feel different as you look at the tree from this distance?

4. Now go even closer so that you are about three feet or one meter from the tree. Anything new that you notice? Look at the detail in the textures, the edges, how one branch flows into another or how the color on one part of the leaf gradually changes hue. How do your eyes feel now about a meter from the tree?

5. Again even closer so your face is just a few centimeters or inches from the tree. Look at the ridges and swirls in the bark. Is the bark on the trunk different from the bark on the branches or is it a smaller version? Notice the texture of a leaf. Trace the edge with your fingers. Feel the bumpiness.

6. Then close your eyes and imagine you are looking through a microscope at the bark or leaf or fruit or blossoms of the tree. What details do you notice? How does the tree feel different to you? How do you feel different?

7. Now reverse the process and back up so you are about three feet or one meter from the tree. What is different from when you were earlier this distance from the tree? Do you notice anything new? Is there a new smell in the air? What has changed?

8. Back up even farther, so you are about 10 feet or three meters from the tree. Do you get a different feeling from the tree? Does the energy around the tree or around you feel different? Calmer? More charged? What feels different?

9. Now back to the starting place 20 feet or seven meters from the tree. Take a good look and notice the details, the variation in the shapes and colors of this individual tree.

10. Finally, Look around yourself. Notice the light. How bright is it? Notice the colors and shapes around you. This is the "after" measurement. Notice where in your body you feel better. How relaxed are your head and shoulders. See whether every part of your body feels comfortable. Take a minute or two to check in with your physical self and your surroundings.

You have just experienced an individual tree, which is unique and yet has a pattern with the various parts of the tree, a smaller or bigger version of each other.

≈≈≈≈≈≈≈

Texture and Elements: Describing Your Way to Better Brain Health

Sensational Medicine, healing the sensory system with new activities. You know the saying, "you can't teach an old dog new tricks. But remember the second half? The fastest way to become an old dog? ... Stop learning new tricks. So in 2013 learn something new, observe a new sensation, notice something old in a new way. These are the ways to improve your brain and eye function. Pick something up every day and notice the shape, color, texture, sound, taste, smell, temperature, consistency, and how the parts make up the whole and how it is connected to its surroundings. How is it similar or different from what is around you?

Blinking exercise like pushups for the eyes. These exercises and more are about 28 minutes into this video Youtube.com/watch?v=JhG3-qwkvVk

≈≈≈≈≈≈≈

Exercise: Describing Your Way To Better Vision

This is a sensory awareness exercise to help you
Sleep deeper
Relax strained eyes
Enjoy more of the beauty around you
Improve peripheral vision

This is also great for people who want to recognize the detail in another person's face and improve relationships.

To use this for relaxation and for people that have trouble sleeping: It's a great exercise to do maybe about half an hour before you want to go to sleep, just to really get yourself present to your sensations and connected to how you feel.

1. In this exercise I would like you to start by looking around yourself, feeling how you feel, what does your body feel like? What do you notice about your surroundings? And just kind of feel your environment,

look at your environment. Notice where you are in time and space.

2. Then pick up an item, a relatively small item that you can hold in your hands. Describe it in as sensory terms as possible. What this means is, describe. Portray the color, the shapes, the size, the texture, and the temperature. Describe the sound of it, the taste of it, and the smell of it? Paint a visual image of it for the listener. Use all your sense to describe it.

What I say to my one-on-one clients is "I should be able to walk in to your house after hearing your description and find the item that you described to me, from your description. I should be able to tell what it is.

For example: I am holding an item. I am going to describe it to you. I am not going to tell you what it is until the end. But, I'm hoping that from my description you will be able to recognize what it is. This item is kind of long and cylindrical and it has a pointy part at one end and a kind of a flat surface at the other end. It is white with kind of a tan design on it. And part of the design has small oval shapes. Along the smooth middle part is some writing and the letters are raised a little bit. So that as I run my finger along the writing on this item, I can feel little bumps. There is also a piece at one end opposite the pointy end, which is a large oval piece. It is a harder, a harder plastic material than the rest of the item. And it is attached by a little ring around the top part of the item. If I tap it, I can hear a sound, that tells me it's kind of a plastic material, and then there is a clicking mechanism that causes the pointy part to go in and out. This doesn't really have a taste; it's not a food item. It doesn't really have a smell. Maybe when it was brand new it might have had a plastic kind of a smell.

And I hope that by now you know that what I had in my hand is a pen, a click pen. That is the kind of detail that I would like you to use to describe. It is best to do it out loud, it doesn't have to be with someone else, but you can call up a friend and say, you know, "Kim gave me this exercise, I have to do. Can I just describe an item to you?"

See if they can guess what the item is from your description of all the different sensations. It doesn't have to be a long time; it can be just a few minutes. Describing something now.

As you noticed it's not just visual information, you're really taking in all the information, through all your five senses. Through your eyes, your ears, taste buds, nose, if it has the appropriate sensations. And certainly touch, and texture, and shape.

Here Is What Researchers Are Saying

"Although there is a vast clinical literature on phantom limbs, there have been no experimental studies on the effects of visual input on phantom sensations. We introduce an inexpensive new device--a 'virtual reality box'--to resurrect the phantom visually to study intersensory effects. A mirror is placed vertically on the table so that the mirror reflection of the patient's intact had is 'superimposed' on the felt position of the phantom. There must be a great deal of back and forth interaction between vision and touch, so that the strictly modular, hierarchical model of the brain that is currently in vogue needs to be replaced with a more dynamic, interactive model, in which 're-entrant' signaling plays the main role." —Ramachandran, V. S. and D. Rogers-Ramachandran (1996). "Synaesthesia in phantom limbs induced with mirrors." *Proc Biol Sci* 263(1369): 377-386.

≈≈≈≈≈≈≈

Exercise: Vision and Visualization

Tibetan eye chart for vision, insight and eyesight. Place the chart with the center line at eye level about an arm's length from your eyes. Moving only your eyes look at each of the outer circles, rotating your eyes in a clockwise direction. Do this twice then do two circle in a counterclockwise direction. Notice the colors and shapes. Then run your eyes through the center from top to bottom, then back to the top again several times. Then run your eyes back and forth a few times along each of the diagonal lines through the center. Notice the patterns, colors and shapes. Next make another circuit around the outer circles clockwise and counter clockwise. Lastly look up to the right, down to the left, up to the left and down to the right creating a figure eight pattern with your eyes.

The chart is at http://kimberlyburnhamphd.com/Self-Care___Intake_Forms.html

≈≈≈≈≈≈≈

Exercise: Color and Sound Therapy

Consider what you are choosing to draw into yourself and your surroundings. What are the colors you are choosing to look at? What colors are you putting on your body every morning? What are the colors of your breakfast? Are you consciously choosing or are you looking, dressing and eating through habit?

In *Color Therapy*, Khwaja Azeemi shares the effect of light, heat and color on cells, organs and on the entire human being. He correlates each organ with a certain color. For example: Heart-Red; Liver-Yellow; Thyroid-Blue; Lungs-Orange; Eyes-Sky Blue; Pancreas-Violet; Phlegmatic Glands (digestive/lymphatic)-Dark Blue; Pituitary Gland-Violet; Spleen-Purple; Bladder-Violet; Testis-Violet; Ovary-Violet.

Would your liver be healthier if you spent more time out in the yellow sunshine, ate more yellow foods with vitamin C or wore yellow socks? What are the colors you are surrounding yourself with and how are those choices influencing your brain health?

Khwaja Azeemi also correlates colors with vitamins: Vitamin A-Yellow; Vitamin B-Green; Vitamin C-Lemon Yellow; Vitamin D-Violet; Vitamin E-Violet; Vitamin K-Dark Blue.

What are you wearing, eating or looking at? What colors surround you? What kind of light are you taking in on a regular basis? Is it the full visual spectrum of sunlight or "junk food" light that strains your eyes?

≈≈≈≈≈≈≈

How Colorful Are Your Goals, Relationships and Life?

With theses exercise many people experience a sense of relaxation, improved eyesight and a greater sense of wellbeing. I would love to hear about your experience. You can contact me through my website: www.KimberlyBurnhamPhD.com.

≈≈≈≈≈≈≈

Part 8: Brain Food: The Sensation of Taste and Smell

Try this exercise for Mindfulness Eating for a better sense of taste, smell and power. For two minutes before eating, stand or sit in the power pose (feet spread wider than shoulders, hands on hips, head up, spine elongated). Think about the food you are about to eat. Think about the temperature, the color, the texture, the shapes, and more. What are you most grateful for? Who prepared the food? Who will you eat it with? Where did it come from?

Thinking about your food—anticipating the food actual makes it easier to digest and absorb the nutrients needed to heal.

≈≈≈≈≈≈

The Disgust Exercises

Next we move to a very different way of thinking about food.

Recognition of the emotion of disgust may save us from eating things that have food poisoning. Awareness of how someone else is responding to us also helps us successfully navigate social situations. For example if I see someone drink sour milk, I see the face they make, perhaps hear the sounds they make and I learn not to eat or drink things that are disgusting and potentially cause food poisoning. I can also see the face of a friend or stranger as they observe me doing something. I can see how they respond. Do they like what I am doing or does it make them uncomfortable? Do they think I am amazing or disgusting? How I interpret their facial features and gestures influences my behavior or I risk being ostracized. From an evolutionary stand point if I eat toxic food or am ostracized from my community I could die.

This emotion or feeling of disgust is intensely personal and often influenced by social and cultural learning. Foods and personal habits that may disgust one person may seem perfectly wonderful to another person. Some things are an acquired taste, where at first it seems disgusting and then gradually becomes more and more appealing.

The ability to have favorite foods or find certain people disgusting and to change those preferences is based in the brain, primarily in a part of the brain called the basal ganglia. This is also the part of the brain that prevents involuntary movements like ticks and tremors.

Imagine a triangle. One side is brain health, particularly the basal ganglia and dopamine function. One side is the emotion of disgust and the third side is voluntary control of movement in the arms and legs as well as the rest of the body.

The emotion of disgust is related to other areas of the brain. It includes the right hemisphere and the negative emotions of sadness, fear, disgust; the amygdala and critical emotions of disgust and indignation; and the insula, which is of central importance for the recognition of disgust and expression of empathy.

≈≈≈≈≈≈≈

Exercise: Disgust—Using the Mind to Heal the Brain

Take about 10 minutes to do this exercise. First, notice how you feel, walk around a little and notice how you are walking, how your balance is, etc. Check in with yourself. Then answer these questions and then re check how you are feeling and notice what has changed.

1. What is the most disgusting food you have ever eaten?
2. What foods do other people like that you find disgusting?
3. What was the last disgusting smell you experienced?
4. What has a disgusting feeling (touch or texture) for you?
5. Whose face did you see with a look of disgust most recently?
6. If you imagine someone offering you something that looks disgusting, how will you respond to them?

You can use these exercises in a similar way to walking. Movement, walking, running and other forms of exercise build your cardiovascular health but they also stimulate your brain to lay down new pathways that become habits. If you walk a mile every morning it feels odd to get up and not walk because you have laid down a pathway in your brain or a habit. Pathways that are often used become stronger. In much the same way you can build new pathways and habits with the disgust exercises. The benefit is that both the walking and the disgust exercise create new pathways in the basal ganglia.

≈≈≈≈≈≈≈

A Princeton post doc characterized these exercises as *"quite brilliant and novel"*. The exercise activates the basal ganglia and insula through noticing what is disgusting. Activating those pathways also improves walking and other functional activities via a different route from practicing motor skills.

"Evermore in the world is this marvelous balance of beauty and disgust, magnificence and rats." —Ralph Waldo Emerson, American Poet, Lecturer and Essayist, 1803-1882

On England and the English: *"As a rule they will refuse even to sample a foreign dish, they regard such things as garlic and olive oil with disgust, life is unlivable to them unless they have tea and puddings"* —George Orwell, English Novelist and Essayist, 1903-1950

≈≈≈≈≈≈≈

A Third Culture Kid's Perspective on Disgusting Foods/Beautiful Truth

Imagine stringy, smelly, fermented soy beans— Japanese natto. Third culture kids, like me have expanded our definition of disgusting foods by traveling widely, sampling mushy grey gruel on the food cars of Chinese trains or sharp pungent onion salad, the only "greens" available on the Trans-Siberian railway or even spoiled key lime pie in Toronto, sitting out in the summer heat, curdling my taste buds.

What disgusting thing have you eaten lately? Come on, we have all eaten disgusting bits of food or even done something disgusting. But did you know, disgust, a beneficial emotion, sometimes saves us from food poisoning and helps us sort out what is true in our lives? And if this is an average day in the United States, thirteen people will die from food poisoning.

In Japan, no one ever says, "yeah, natto it is okay. I am fine with or without it." You either hate it or, and I can't understand this part, love it. Seriously, there are people whose favorite food is brown, slimy natto. It's super healthy for your heart but only if you can keep it down.

"Sushi," explains, my father, an avid fisherman, "has an English translation—bait." And yet there are millions of people worldwide who love fresh raw tuna.

Me, I can't stand the feel of it sliding down my throat, even after four years in Japan.

Global travelers or Third Culture Kids like me have also experienced some of the loveliest foods in the world. It has been nearly fifty years; I still remember the sweet creamy texture of a tree-ripened mango in Bogota, Colombia. Sitting atop a slippery slide in our walled backyard, juice dripped down my chin, staining my blue and white checked shirt. With my teeth, I scraped off every last bit of yellow-orange flesh before following the big white pit down the slide and running inside for another mango.

We value certain foods much higher than others, with a part of the brain called the basal ganglia, part of the subcortical brain, the basal ganglia also forms a link between goal directed behavior and habit forming rewards. Goal driven, we can seek out new foods, new experiences or habitually order our favorite foods in restaurants. Maybe we are addicted to certain foods. Researchers call this a maladaptive type of habit learning or maybe we have an appetitive Pavlovian conditioning to certain foods we grew up with, driven by the limbic system part of the brain.

What is your favorite food? Do you have a favorite restaurant where you always order the same thing? Do you try different kinds of foods at home or in new restaurants?

Think of your brain influenced food choices, as bright yellow buses on a highway. You can achieve your goals and get where you are going, on whichever one you want. You get to choose. By choosing wisely, you improve the journey, the road, and become more functional. Choose unwisely and you will get food poisoning or ostracized from the community.

In the same way that walking and taking fish oils improves brain function, consciously noticing what disgusts or excites you can lay down shiny new neural pathways and create memories that last a lifetime.

Pattern recognition skills needed to experience and identify disgust in the faces of others is compromised in people with brain dysfunctions like depression, Huntington's disease (a genetic movement disorder), focal dystonia (unusually tight twisted muscles), Parkinson's disease (tremor movement disorder), and Wilson's disease (genetic copper processing disorder).

Consciously considering what is disgusting is one way to help heal the brain. Think of disgust exercises as weight training for your brain.

In addition to your brain's culinary ability, researchers Sam Harris, et al in 2008 Annals of Neurology note another function of the basal ganglia.

"The difference between believing and disbelieving a proposition is one of the most potent regulators of human behavior and emotion." Whether we accept something as true or reject it as a false string of words, depends on the health of our brain. Continuing he says, "Truth may be beauty, and beauty truth, in more than a metaphorical sense, and false propositions may actually disgust us."

For a few years in the 1980's I couldn't eat anything that tasted like mango because in Malaysia, I got sick drinking mango flavored water.

Now, my rational mind knew it was probably some contamination in the water not the mango powder but my body carried a powerful memory of the last thing I drank before starting to throw up. I literally couldn't even smell a mango without that nauseas feeling coming back.

It was compounded by the fact that I was on vacation on Tioman Island, Malaysia with a wicked bad sunburn, throwing up sick, no appetite for spicy, the-only-food-available, sleeping in a little hut on the beach with sand and who knows what else in the sheets, and an Asian style squatty potty a ways down the beach. But, I still remember the beautiful sunsets and my girlfriend looking at me and saying, with a laugh, "Just think, people at home are envying us."

≈≈≈≈≈≈≈

Part 9: Movement Therapies and Parkinson's

Move it or lose it! Here is some of what the research is saying about the benefits of movement therapies for people with Parkinson's disease.

Today you can find practitioners and instructors of movement therapies such as Qigong, Taichi, Yoga, Pilates, and more in many places from private clinics, hospitals and physical therapy clinics to gyms and dance studios. Many public recreation facilities and schools also have movement therapy classes available.

Qigong

In a study of Qigong, an ancient Chinese psychosomatic [mind-body] exercise, research found that the integrated movement, breathing and meditation had an effect on mood and subjective sleep quality. In other words, practitioners had enhanced psychological well-being, including sleep duration. —Manzaneque, J. M., F. M. Vera, et al. (2009). "Serum cytokines, mood and sleep after a qigong program: is qigong an effective psychobiological tool?" *J Health Psychol* 14(1): 60-67. [Medline Abstract].

Yoga, Taichi and Qigong Improves Balance and Gait

In an investigation of the effect of regular Qigong exercise on Parkinson's symptoms, researchers noted "Qigong is an exercise therapy based on the principles of Traditional Chinese Medicine. The exercises combine the practice of motion and rest, both guided by mental imagery. The movements or postures are thought to promote an "energy flow" along meridians, which are not related to anatomic structures." They reported a beneficial effect of Qigong for gait imbalances and joint problems.

The Qigong exercises used in their study "can be classified as active physiotherapy using low-energy exercises with sustained movements of limbs, trunk, face and tongue as well as breathing coordination and can be adapted to special needs." —Schmitz-Hübsch, T., D. Pyfer, et al. (2006). "Qigong exercise for the symptoms of PD: a randomized, controlled pilot study." *Mov Dis* 21(4):543. from www.ncbi.nlm.nih.gov

Six months of a combination of Taichi and Qigong training improved the balance in 33 healthy older adults compared to 16 others in a wait-list control —Yang Y, Verkuilen JV, Rosengren KS et al: Effect of combined Taiji and Qigong training on balance mechanisms: a randomized controlled trial of older adults. *Med Sci Monit*, 2007; 13(8): CR339–48.

While evaluating the changes in sensory and biomechanical balance mechanisms, it was inferred that

Taichi-Qigong improves balance through better vestibular [ears and temporal lobe] inputs and wider stance.

Yoga is another Asian practice which was shown to improve the hip extension, increase the stride length and decrease anterior pelvic tilt, hence improving the gait in older people. —[DiBenedetto M, Innes KE, Taylor AG et al: Effect of a gentle Iyengar yoga program on gait in the elderly: an exploratory study. *Arch Phys Med Rehabil*, 2005; 86(9): 1830–37].

In another randomized controlled trial 69 older persons were randomly allocated to three groups i.e., Yoga, Ayurveda (herbal) and a Wait-list control group. There were 23 subjects in each group (with seven males in the Yoga group and six males each in Ayurveda and Wait-list control groups).

All three groups had comparable baseline values with respect to measures of gait and balance as well as mobility.

At the end of six months, the Yoga group (18 people at follow-up) showed a significant increase in the overall scores for gait and balance.

For The Up and Go Test (TUG) [a commonly used walking assessment] both Yoga and Ayurveda groups showed a significant decrease in the number of steps taken to complete the test. This means the stride length increases. This is significant in Parkinson's disease because a short shuffling gait or way of walking is typical as the disease process progresses. This research indicates that movement therapies can slow or stop the progression and add to improvements. It is important to note that in what is thought to be a progressive disease; even just stopping the progression of the symptoms is a significant improvement.

Normal gait and balance depends on several factors including free joint mobility, appropriate timing and intensity of muscle action as well as normal sensory input.

Yoga practice improved the joint mobility in rheumatoid arthritis patients. —Haslock I, Monro R, Nagarathna R et al: Measuring the effects of yoga in rheumatoid arthritis. *Br J Rheumatol,* 1994; 33(8): 788].

In persons with normal health there was an improvement in the muscle strength. —[Raghuraj P, Nagarathna R, Nagendra HR et al: Pranayama increases grip strength without lateralized effects. *Indian J Physiol Pharmacol,* 1997; 41(2): 129–33]—visual perceptual sensitivity and the ability to balance on a stabilometer.

The changes in the present study may be attributed to the beneficial effects of yoga mentioned above, while the changes in the Ayurveda group could be related to improved muscle strength and better sensory perception as hypothesized in traditional Ayurveda texts. —[Shastri P: Sharangadhara Samhita, Adhamalla teeka. *Varanasi: Oriental Publishers & Distributors,* 1985] and Krishnamurthy, M. and S. Telles (2007). "Effects of Yoga and an Ayurveda preparation on gait, balance and mobility in older persons." *Med Sci Monit* 13(12): LE19-20.

~~~~~~~

Exercise: Participate in a Movement Therapy Class

1. Ask friends or family members or health care professionals about movement therapies they have tried or that they recommend.

2. Try out a class or a series of classes.

3. Notice what changes in your walking, your flexibility, your energy levels and how comfortable you are moving and functioning.

Part 10: Conclusion

The very best way to know if these techniques and self-care exercises will help you is to pick one. This about which one will be easiest or the most fun for you to do. Do you like to do things alone or in a group? Do you want to start by visualizing the exercises or jump in physically?

It is never too soon to start feeling better.

≈≈≈≈≈≈≈

Exercise: Pick One

1. Pick one exercise in this book.

2. Do it daily for a week.

3. Notice what changes in your walking, your flexibility, your energy levels and how comfortable you are moving and functioning.

4. Continue to do the same exercise or pick a new one to do or add an exercise to do for the next week.

≈≈≈≈≈≈≈

About the Author: Kimberly Burnham, PhD, The Nerve Whisperer

Passionate about changing the face of brain health worldwide, I continue to do everything I can to get out a message of hope, practical solutions for conditions from sleep disturbances, insomnia, chronic pain, migraines, and memory loss to traumatic brain injuries, Parkinson's disease, Huntington's, ALS and autism.

My message is supported by a PhD in Integrative Medicine (2006) with my dissertation topic, *The Effect of Integrative Manual Therapy on Symptoms of Parkinson's Disease*. I am also happy to share my own story of recovery from migraines and vision issues and powerful examples of improved quality of life from the thousands of clients I have worked with over the last 15 years. I specialize in finding solutions for people with a diagnosis of Parkinson's disease, macular degeneration, multiple sclerosis, Huntington's ataxia, Lyme's disease and other brain and nervous system issues.

I believe, what we expect and observe, influences what we get. People in my practice can expect my full attention as well as positive changes and progress with their goals. It is best to come to the first session having thought about your goals. If anything, truly anything, can shift about your health, your life, your relationships, your way of being in the world, what do you want? What does "better" look and feel like for you.

I have treatment sessions available at St Luke's Rehabilitation Institute in Spokane, Washington (509) 473-6869 and often do phone or skype consulting with clients world-wide.

Physical therapists, chiropractors, naturopaths, acupuncturists and other health-care practitioners may contact me for work in your clinic for a week or so at a time, anywhere in the world. Please contact me at theburnhamreview@juno.com if I can help support your individual healing or clinical practice.

≈≈≈≈≈≈≈

Work with Kimberly Burnham, PhD Today

Do You Need a Speaker for Your Next Conference?

I speak at large conferences, small focus groups, online summits and radio shows. Please contact me so I can help your audience members or clients live with less pain and more success. Here is a replay of my presentation at the *Global Raising Consciousness Now Summit* at http://consciousnessnow.tv/video/interview-with-kimberly-burnham-phd-on-the-2012-consciousness-raising-summit. It is also available on YouTube at http://www.youtube.com/watch?v=JhG3-qwkvVk

Inspirational as well as step-by-step self-help books can be found on my Amazon Author's Page at www.amazon.com/Kimberly-Burnham/e/B0054RZ4A0

Please see my LinkedIn profile for a selection of upcoming presentations and clinical consultations at http://www.linkedin.com/in/kimberlyburnham

I would love to speak to your book club, health related gathering, or train you on the value of diversity, vision recovery, Parkinson's solutions, improving symptoms in genetic diagnoses, and more. Please contact me at TheBurnhamReview@juno.com or (860) 221-8510 US PST (Spokane, WA) to set up an in-person presentation or skype meeting. I also do a number of guest blogs every month.

≈≈≈≈≈≈≈

www.ingramcontent.com/pod-product-compliance
Lightning Source LLC
Chambersburg PA
CBHW070924270326
41927CB00011B/2708